DEDICATION

I dedicate this book to every living being out there who is suffering with physical, mental, or emotional pain and illness. There is HOPE.

ACKNOWLEDGEMENTS

I would first like to thank my mentor and health consultant Aajonus Vonderplanitz for the important work he did during his time here. It is because of Aajonus that this book exists.

Next, I would like to thank my mother for instilling confidence and perseverance, and for teaching me to always have an open mind. These are three of the greatest gifts that you have given me and for this I am forever grateful.

Thank you to my dad and Lorraine for all of your support through the challenging times towards the end of the release of this book. You were always there when I needed a pick-me-up.

Thank you to my family…aunt Peggy for providing your home and a warm bed to stay during my writing of this book, and to aunt Wanda and to all of my cousins for always supporting me through all of my crazy ideas.

Thank you to Eaden Shantay for guiding me into the direction of alternative ways. I grew up with the knowing of only conventional western medicine and did not even know there were other options out there until our meeting. Thank you for showing me new ways.

And last, but certainly not least, I want to thank my daughter Sedona who is truly the love of my life and for whom I hope to always be a positive role model. You were the reason I dove head first into researching how food impacts the body.

Thank you to Source and all of the unseen angels in my life.

raw to

radiant

the secrets to a long life of

radiant health

by Kimberly Lynn Williams

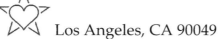

Radiant Health Publishing.

Los Angeles, CA 90049

Cover Design by: Lynnette Greenfield
Cover Layout: Josh Dery
Photography by: Victoria Griggs, Sedona Cohen, and other unnamed photographers.
Graphics: Andrej Semnic

INTRODUCTION

The purpose of this book is to provide you with information on how to live a long healthy life. It has been proven that the primary cause of disease is from exposure to environmental poisons. This book provides scientifically documented information that is not readily spoken about or marketed by mainstream media on how to rid the body of these toxins, reversing disease and chronic illness. We have created these poisons ourselves that are slowly kill us, our children, and the world we live in, although lately it seems we are doing it much more quickly.

I am not here to preach to you, but rather to heighten your awareness of what we are doing to create the diseases we live with and to provide you with an alternative to improving your physical well-being. It is to make you aware of the choices you make each day so that maybe you can change one thing that can lead you toward a healthier life. Bringing your awareness to what you are putting into your body will facilitate small changes now that may lead to bigger changes in the future. I ask you to have an open mind and think "out of the box" when reading this book. It has come to you because you are ready at some level for this information.

I will inform you of the choices you have when it comes to treating ailments; specifically, how certain foods support the detoxification and healing process in the body. I believe the human body is designed to heal itself of nearly every ailment if we remove the poisons that create the problem and rebuild the body. There is a tremendous amount of scientific evidence on this subject which I present here.

Our aging population is growing faster than ever before. Take control of your health. Free yourself of disease and slow down the aging process now!

AUTHOR'S NOTE

I feel it is important to share my background and experiences that guided my food transitions through my life as my story is that of a very ordinary person in which most people can relate. I was born and raised in the Flint, Michigan. The only child of a single mother, I spent ample time at my grandparent's house where my grandmother cooked traditional meals and where most everything was fried in bacon grease. In fact, there was always a tin can of it sitting on the stove, ready for the hot skillet. Junk food, as we know it, was just starting to make its way into our home and I was a big fan of processed cereals, and Hostess Ding Dongs.

At about age seven, I was old enough to be home alone after school while my mom worked. As a latch key kid, most of my meals were either TV dinners cooked in aluminum; toaster or microwave meals, or fast food. It was cheap and it was not uncommon to have had to hunt for loose change in coat pockets or in the sofa on the days before payday to find enough money to pay for a burger from the local fast food joint. Nothing out of the ordinary for a kid of a single working mother living in Flint.

I will leap ahead to college where my diet consisted mostly of canned Spaghetti O's, white bread, saltines with peanut butter and jelly, and salads. I was a dancer and gymnast, modeled, and competed in the local and state Miss America Organization scholarship pageants to earn scholarship money for college. Keeping my weight down was crucial and a constant struggle. No matter what I ate, I always felt bloated and was one of those people that had to work out several hours a day, nearly seven days a week to just maintain my weight. It seemed that along with exercise, my caloric intake had to be extremely low, like 500 – 600 calories a day, just to lose a few pounds. I now understand how the high carb/grain diet negatively impacted my body.

When I graduated from college, I was hired by one of the largest pharmaceutical companies in the world to sell prescription pharmaceuticals and pediatric vaccinations. I was later recruited by medical companies and transitioned into medical device sales. I sold electromagnetic frequency bone-growth stimulators that treated broken bones and spinal fusions that would not heal, titanium and stainless-steel rods/plates and screws for spinal reconstruction, knee braces, and heart catheters. I spent about 10 years as a medical sales rep in southern Michigan and made good money which allowed me to eat high quality food and meals at nice restaurants.

In my mid-thirties, I left the industry to start my family. My daughter was born with severe food allergies to dairy, soy, corn, and wheat. I had a difficult time finding treats that tasted good that she did not have a reaction to, so I created *Idella's Natural Gourmet*, a cookie company that produced gourmet organic cookies free of wheat, dairy, soy and corn. At the same time, I began studying nutrition and the healing effects of specific foods on the body.

During my studies, I learned how most ailments as we know them are really forms of either an over poisoning of the body from environmental exposures, or a detoxification process of the body. I also learned how bacteria and viruses do not make us sick, but are actually designed to detoxify us. This information was a bit shocking as it was the complete opposite of everything I had learned growing up and yet there was something about what I was reading that felt right.

While studying the health benefits of raw foods, I learned about how the toxic effects of specific cooked foods, especially heated nut and seed oils impact the body in a destructive way. My conscious got me...How could I continue selling and making money from cookies, knowing they were contributing to disease? I discontinued my cookie business and opened an organic raw food storefront where I sold everything raw. This was NOT a raw vegan store. We made sushi, ceviche', carpaccio, beef/tuna tartare dishes, fresh raw coconut cream, raw fruit & vegetable juices, smoothies, and raw nuts/seeds and their oils. I was also a pick-up location and delivery person for the local raw dairy in our community in the Aspen, Colorado valley where residents could get fresh raw unpasteurized farm milk straight from the cow, the way nature intended.

Although I will refer to raw unheated foods frequently in this book, you will see that I have found that it is not necessary to be on a 100% raw diet to have change happen in the body, although it is not uncommon for people who have struggled with very serious illnesses to "go for it" so to speak to turn around their ailments, or prevent their own death from cancer, and then be able to gradually add some cooked food back into their diet. I will however, address how much raw food is believed to be necessary each day to pull poisons from the body. I have learned that there are incredible dishes that can be made with raw meats such as Wild Salmon Ceviche' made with a red onion, jalapeno, tomato, avocado and cilantro sauce.

It is also important to note that I am not promoting a vegan diet of sprouting, soaking and dehydrating nuts and seeds trying to make them appear as pizza. This works well for some people, but I personally do not have the genetic mutation that allows me to eat a 100% vegan diet and survive well, nor do a large amount of people on the planet. Cornell University found a vegetarian allele (vegetarian gene) that allows some people to survive on a vegetarian diet alone without needing to eat animal protein. One of their studies showed that as of 2018, only 18% of Americans actually have this vegetarian gene. The rest of us need some form of animal protein to survive well or our health declines. This explained why some vegans would come to me for assistance when their health deteriorated, and why the Dali Lama had to add animal protein to his diet to survive. Well-meaning parents feed babies plant-based milks but if the baby does not have the genetics to be a vegetarian this can be extremely detrimental for the developing brain and body of a child. Once again, let's think about this logically....babies are humans and humans are animals and we were designed to consume animal (human) milk.

This book is a roadmap to health through food and gives you information on specific food categories and then allows you to choose which foods work best for YOUR body and it works for everyone whether you eat meat, are vegetarian, vegan, pescatarian, primal, paleo, etc. Incorporating these concepts has changed my life personally. It is one of the main factors that allows me to maintain a healthy fit weight, along with exercise, and a positive mental attitude. I do not fear eating fat any longer, I do not fear bacteria and viruses any longer, and I no longer fear disease any longer.

THE WORLD WE LIVE IN

Whatever your belief.... The creation of the earth by God or the science of evolution, it really makes no difference. The world we were created to live in is a world of nature and we were designed to live in this nature with nature.

In this vast world in which we live, there are many different kinds of biomes. The oceans and lakes are their own biomes, the rainforest is its own biome, the deserts are each their own biome, a grassy savanna is its own biome, and the arctic tundra would be its own biome. Each of these areas have specific creatures that survive within it. And within each biome are microbiomes or micro-worlds that are made up of microscopic organisms, viruses, parasites and molds.

The human body is no different. We are also made up of microscopic organisms, viruses, parasites and molds. In fact, there are 100 Trillion microbes that live in and on every person. There are also more than 10,000 different microbial species that researchers have identified so far, living in and on the human body. Our world is made up of worlds within worlds within worlds within a world. And we are all designed for all of this to work synergistically together.

bi-ome: *noun* - a naturally occurring community of flora and microbes.

We are designed to live synergistically with bacteria and viruses and have lived this way for millions of years.

And then one day all of a sudden we were told that these microbes were dangerous and that now we are going to call them "GERMS" because they make us sweat, and have fevers, and throw up, and have diarrhea, and get rashes, and make us cough up phlegm and mucus and give us stomach aches, and that you should be afraid. Very afraid. Very, very afraid.

WHAT?!?!?! We have lived in nature with microbes for billions and billions of years and suddenly they are our enemies? This is completely illogical and yet this is what is and has been taught in medical schools for decades. The truth is that what we call "germs" are not actually the "cause" of disease, but they actually act like little super-heros in our body and in our world. Bacteria, viruses, parasites, and molds are designed to break down toxins, decayed cells, dead cells and debris in and on our body. Our body naturally uses these microbes to reduce its toxicity level to a smaller amount so it can eliminate these toxins and debris very efficiently. The actual elimination of the debris in our body is the "symptoms" that we experience.

The human body is amazing and is naturally designed to move out toxins and debris. The most efficient way for the body to rid itself of poisons is to vomit it out. An example of this is when a person drinks too much alcohol. If the body does not respond efficiently to the consumption of an over-abundance of alcohol by throwing up, that individual can get alcohol poisoning and die very quickly. Diarrhea is another way the body eliminates poisons super efficiently. The body dumps toxins and debris into the stomach and moves it out through the GI tract as quickly as it can so the toxins do not do too much damage on their way out. It brings fluids to the area to flush them out fast. In addition to vomit and diarrhea, breath, urine, tears, ear wax, nasal discharge, phlegm, rashes, hives, and sweat, are all ways that poisons and debris escape the human body.

Germ Theory: Louis Pasteur is best known for formulating the germ theory. His idea was that an outside organism (a germ) would enter a human body, wreaking havoc on their system. He believed that these "germs" were monomorphic, meaning they have only one form and are non-changeable, although he was never able to prove his theory and we have since learned that this is actually not true.

There is much controversy written about Pasteur and his methods and it is said that many were not properly carried out and many more unscientific. For example, in one study, Pasteur injected the blood of one sick animal into a healthy animal making the animal sick. He concluded that it was the germ from the sick animal that made the healthy animal ill, but he forgot to take into account what else may have been in that blood that was transferred to the animal and may have contributed to the illness. Also, one can be exposed to a germ and still not have the symptoms of the illness while another person exposed to the same germ and that has a toxic body can have the symptoms.

Around the same time as Pasteur, a contemporary of his, Antoine Bechamp, was finding no truth to the germ theory in his research. In fact, he and many other colleagues were able to prove quite the opposite, that cells contained molecular granulations which he called "microzyma" and Gunther Enderlein called endobionts (Greek for bios-life). These microorganisms live inside us and unlike cells, are virtually indestructible. They are pleomorphic, meaning they can change into many different forms as needed. These microorganisms have been seen under the microscope to morph from a microbe to bacteria to a fungus to a virus. Dr. Robert Young, author of the book "Sick and Tired", reports viewing a red blood cell turn into a bacterium and then back into a red blood cell again. The microzyma or endobionts morph into whatever form the body needs to breakdown toxins and debris in the body. The terrain or environment of the body determines what form they take.

I am not saying that it is not possible to obtain an outside organism, but one will not experience a detoxification or cleansing from it unless your body needs it (at least not a cleansing that is noticeable). We all come in contact with hundreds, maybe thousands, of bacteria and organisms every day and yet we do not get sick every day. That is why Pasteur's germ theory does not hold up. Many people with a particular disease show no signs of having a specific germ that caused that disease. And, many healthy individuals have shown signs of so called "pathogenic germs".

But what about the "Black Plague" that swept across Europe killing so many? One can trace every illness back to environmental poisoning and deficiencies. During the time of plagues, homes were heated by burning toxic substances. Coal was one of them. What does coal release into the air when burned? Mercury; one of the most toxic elements on the planet. These people were already poisoned. A bacteria was created to detoxify their body but they did not understand at this time how to rebuild the body as it was detoxing, so death occurred.

This is why I asked you to be open and think "outside of the box". Pasteur's unproven works took off like wildfire while the important works of Bechamp, Naessen and Enderlein were lost in the feeding frenzy of vaccinations, pharmaceuticals and the big business of the "germ theory". The health care industry's basis on the germ theory has created one of the biggest industries in the world. The mega food industry is right up there with it, due to the fact that what we ingest affects the terrain of our body causing a need for the "germs" to feed on the debris and poisons, in its effort to try to save us. More on this to come.

Today's physicians are only preaching what they have been taught in their "books of knowledge". In order for them to practice medicine they must not deviate away from what they had to memorize for their exams or question the germ theory that they were taught. I believe that they either truly believe what they are doing is true and beneficial, or they are too afraid to question the authority that is over them or they will lose their license to practice. Fortunately, alternative methods are making their way back into healing centers, while integrative medicine which combines both conventional western medicine with alternative medicine, is in high demand these days.

WHERE IS THE EVIDENCE?

How do we know this to be true? What happens when you pick a piece of fruit off a tree and let is sit for too long? It begins to die. What happens when it dies? It grows mold on it. The once healthy cells deteriorate and die, and the mold grows on these cells to break them down to get rid of them. If you have ever left some produce in the refrigerator drawer just a little too long you know that bacteria and mold can develop and break down that once living food into pretty much nothing but water if you leave it there long enough. Now the produce did not leave your refrigerator and come in contact with some bacteria and mold in the outside world and then make its way back to your refrigerator drawer. The cells started to die, and the produce created its own bacteria and mold to help it breakdown.

Leeches, maggots and other parasites have been used for centuries to clean out debris and decay from wounds. Today they are called "medicinal parasites" and are even being used in upscale spas in facial treatments to eat away dead skin cells, kind of like how an acid peel would work without the risk of chemicals on the skin absorbing into healthy cells. There are even oil-eating microbes that consume toxic petroleum and have been used in oil spills to assist in clean-up.

Every living thing has a way of cleaning up its own garbage. Watch a pile of compost decompose. Mold, parasites and bacteria do their jobs to break down the dead materials. Inside the body, bacteria, viruses, parasites and molds do exactly the same thing. They breakdown the bad stuff to assist us in its removal and there are many studies from top medical institutions from all over the world to prove this.

Oncolytic viral therapy is a medical treatment that uses viruses to treat cancer and started being used when it was discovered that cancer tumors regressed after a patient went through a viral "illness" such as when they got the flu. Viruses have been used since at least 1912 when the rabies virus was injected into patients to treat cancer of the cervix.

- Harvard Medical School used the herpes virus to destroy brain tumors.
- Swiss researchers injected colon cancer cells with a virus and eliminated the cancer. They noted that "viruses could damage cancer cells while sparing normal cells".
- Researchers from Stanford University, The Mayo Clinic in Rochester, MN and the M.D. Anderson Cancer Center in Houston injected the common cold virus into patients with gastrointestinal cancer that had spread to the liver. The patient's tumors shrank and those receiving the highest dose of the virus lived the longest. They noted no risk besides having mild flu like symptoms.
- Korean scientists injected salmonella into metastasized tumors stopping tumor growth and metastasis prolonging survival and with no side effects.

- Researchers at MIT and University of California San Diego injected salmonella into cancerous tumors reducing and eliminating them.
- As reported in the New York Times, Dr. James Arseneau, at Albany Medical Center is testing the injection of a virus into advanced head and neck cancer patients with "superb results".
- A study published in Nature Medicine shows how a team at Harvard Medical School injected brain tumors with the herpes virus enabling the virus to destroy the tumors.
- Typically, most patients with Glioma, an aggressive form of brain tumor, die within one year. "This treatment is more effective than anything we have done before" says Antonio Chiocca, Harvard Medical School associate professor of surgery at Massachusetts General Hospital.
- Scientists from Calgary and London, Ontario have used a poxvirus to completely destroy human brain tumors in mice. The poxvirus showed in the tumor but did not spread to other parts of the body.
- Yale University proved that Salmonella bacterium reduced solid cancerous tumors in mice. Vion Pharmaceuticals is doing current testing on humans with a drug called Tapet that is an attenuated form of Salmonella because there is evidence that salmonella scavenges the body of degenerative and toxic tissue.
- Cultures all over the world eat salmonella on a regular basis to cleanse and detoxify.

- In 2015 the first double-mutated herpes virus was approved in the United States to treat melanoma.
- Scientists have proven that parts of the world where intestinal parasites exist, IBD and Crohn's rarely exists.

In most of medicine, doctors give patients pills to counter what is happening in their body. They are not in pain because they are deficient of pain medication. They are not experiencing high blood pressure because they are deficient in beta-blockers or diuretics. They do not have asthma or arthritis because they are deficient in steroids. However, medicine has this one right by using viral therapy. Cancer is caused because a person is deficient in viruses (or bacteria). However, you don't have to take a bacteria or virus pill to destroy your cancer. Cancer happens when toxins and cellular debris do not get cleansed out of the body so a cocoon, or capsule forms around them which we call a tumor. Instead of needing bacteria and virus pills to treat the tumors by breaking down the cocoon and dead cells, why not let natural bacteria and viruses treat them the way they were designed to? Or better yet, prevent the tumors from forming in the first place.

Bacteria and viruses are nature's way of breaking down toxins and degenerative cellular debris so our body can move it out as efficiently as possible preventing you from getting cancerous tumors. Is the key not prevention? Why would you want to be a statistic? We were naturally designed to detoxify with the help of these micro-organisms. Stopping the detoxification stops the natural cleansing of your body. The reason one individual may get extremely ill and have an intense detoxification is because one, they have a tremendous amount of toxic build-up in their body to clean out and two, they keep putting more toxins in their body giving the microbes more to feed on. The key to health is to rebuild new healthy cells during the detoxification process. So while you are cleaning out the old dead cells, you are rebuilding new healthy cells.

The bulk of adverse genetic mutations are created in one person's lifetime from the toxic choices they make, not from inheritance. Of course, once the genetic alteration has happened, they can then pass that mutated gene to their offspring. Then that offspring continues toxic choices that can create additional genetic mutations. This pattern is highly destructive unless changes are made.

THE CAUSE OF DISEASE AND CHRONIC ILLNESS

If germs are not the cause of disease and chronic illness, then what is? The truth is, there are two primary causes:

1. environmental poisons and,
2. deficiencies.

We were designed to live in this world......

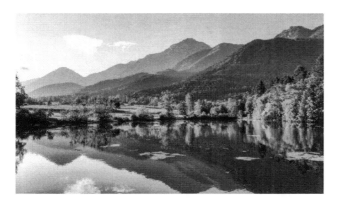

Not this world...

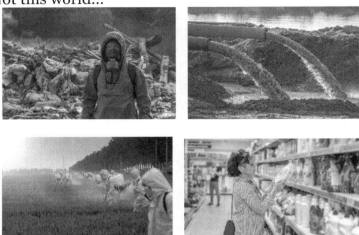

There are over 80,000 chemicals used in the United States but unfortunately relatively few have actually been tested for their effects on the human body. In addition to chemicals, there are physical toxins that have a physical impact on healthy cells as well causing destruction. Examples of these kinds of toxins include: x-rays, mammograms, MRI's, ultrasounds, CT scans, as well as the electromagnetic pollution from microwaves, cell phones, phone towers, electrical transformers and other electronic sources.

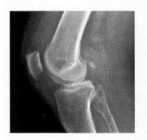
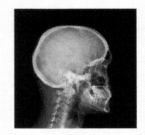

HOW CHEMICAL TOXINS CAUSE DISEASE

When chemicals enter the body, they can damage or completely destroy healthy cells in their path. Some toxins get flushed out naturally with body fluids, while some store extracellularly on the outside of cells or in between cells and some store inside cells weakening them. Some cells get completely destroyed as toxins move through the body. There is a great video created by the University of Calgary showing how brain cells grow and how mercury not only stops the growth but dissolves them instantly. Isolated live snail brain cells are shown growing in a petri dish and the tiniest drop of mercury is deposited into the dish. You can watch the brain cells disintegrate right before your eyes. The scientists explain how snail brain cell growth cones are virtually identical in all animals including man. This is a powerful example of heavy metal damage that happens in our brain contributing to neurological diseases such as dementia.

Some toxins make their way into the bloodstream where they circulate around the body about once every minute. As they circulate through the brain, vital organs and tissues, they can cause additional cellular death in their path leaving what we call cellular debris or cell corpses.

Again, our body is designed to naturally detoxify itself, so it is trying to get these poisons out as quickly and efficiently as possible. The problem is that we have created a world where we are exposed to environmental poisons nearly every moment of every day of our lives causing there to be more toxins and dead cells in our body than can be removed naturally. When enough healthy cells have been destroyed in a particular part of the body, and those cells can no longer be replaced mostly due to poor diet, that body part stops functioning the way it was designed to function and medical professionals give it a name. This is what we call "disease". So if sugar and other toxins destroy a pancreas we label this "diabetes". If toxins damage healthy cells in the G.I. tract while moving out the body causing inflammation and ulcers, we call this colitis or ulcerative colitis. When alcohol and poisons damage healthy cells of the liver we call this cirrhosis. When environmental poisons damage brain cells causing interruptions of neuro connections, we call this Autism, Dementia or Alzheimer's. When toxins damage the lining of arteries causing cooked oil toxins to store and accumulate there preventing blood flow, we call this Atherosclerosis. When poisons damage the myelin sheath of the nerve cells in the brain causing loss of motor skills, convulsions, loss of concentration we label this ALD. When environmental poisons store in and damage the appendix, it brings fluids to that area trying to flush the toxins out inflaming that area and we have appendicitis. Toxic waste collects in the eyes of some people and we call these cataracts. When toxins, waste and dead cells are not moved out of the body, the body goes into protection mode by forming a capsule or tomb around the waste and toxins. This is how a tumor is created and is what causes cancer.

Nearly every ailment can be attributed to environmental poisons and deficiencies causing damage to healthy cells to an area of the body. Stay out in the sun too long and you cook your skin cells killing them. We call this a sunburn. If you do it too many times for too long of a time you can do permanent damage to your organ called "the skin" or cause premature aging as the skin deteriorates. This is the exact same thing that happens to organs that are inside your body. Too much damage to an organ from all of the environmental poisons you are exposed to and that organ stops functioning well, especially if there are toxins and dead cells clogging up the organ. Just cleaning out an organ of dead cells can help jump start its engine again. Add to that the rebuilding of new healthy cells and you can get parts working again that you did not think could work again.

You can see now that a "bacterial infection" or a "viral infection" is actually a detoxification that our body is going through and the symptoms are actually the toxins coming out. But what do we do? Instead of allowing these natural detoxifications to happen, we stop them with medications like antibiotics which kill the bacteria, stopping the detox and keeping the toxins and dead cells in the body while adding more poisons, thus creating a greater buildup of debris in our body. Nature, wanting to do what it is designed to do does not understand why the bacteria it created to breakdown the toxins and debris did not work (because you took the antibiotics to destroy the bacteria). At some point, the body says, "ok, I have tried these bacteria several times now and they are not doing what they need to do so I am going to create a stronger one to do the trick". This is what we call a "super bug" or an antibiotic resistant bacterium.

We were put on this planet to live synergistically with nature. I am not saying I am opposed to modern medicine. The creation of modern medicines and technologies are incredible and there is a place for them. I have and will use them as needed. But the pendulum has swung too far in one direction and we have gotten too far away from our true nature. The combination of stopping these natural detoxifications, the addition of medication residues, and all of the pollutants that we are exposed to on a daily basis, has created a toxic body overload. The problem is that we are exposed too many poisons that are creating too much damage and debris in our body, and then we are preventing our body from eliminating them thus they turn into cancer or some other form of debilitating illness.

DIFFERENT KINDS OF TOXINS

It is important to understand that we are exposed to environmental poisons nearly 24/7/365 and that there is no longer any place in the world that you can go where you will not be impacted by them to some degree. Understanding the different kinds and categories of environmental poisons and becoming aware of what is damaging to your physical body is essential so you can increase your awareness and pick your poisons.

We all have choices that we are not willing to give up. I am not asking a professional golfer to give up his game of golf because he breathes in some level of pesticides, herbicides and chemicals that are used to keep the golf courses pristine, but he/she CAN make the choice to cut out other poisons in his/her life, especially those which are breathed in such as caustic household cleaners. A professional hair colorist is exposed to some pretty toxic chemicals every day as well, but if it's their life, their passion, they are not going to walk away from something they love. However, they can add air purifiers to their salon, and make other choices to reduce their toxic body load. These are just two examples. There are not many jobs in the world today that do not increase the poison load of the physical body. Later I will discuss how you can incorporate food that detoxifies your body of the poisons you are exposed to each day.

When I talk about toxins, most people usually think of industrial chemicals. As I mentioned earlier, we are exposed to an enormous amount of chemicals, both natural and man-made which are extremely detrimental to our health. They are in our water, our food, our soil, our air, in the beds we sleep in, the vehicles we drive, the offices we work in, the stores we shop in, in schools, on the playgrounds, etc. In addition to chemicals, there are also physical toxins such as x-rays, ultrasound, mammography, MRI's, CT's, as well as microwave radiation, gamma rays, ultraviolet light, and electro-magnetic frequency such as with cell phones and cell towers. These physical toxins impact the body as well destroying healthy cells and leaving cellular debris and cell corpses inside of us.

Stress
Stress can also have an impact on healthy cells in your body both directly and indirectly. There are mental toxins, emotional toxins, energetic toxins, and toxic communication, all of which can again do physical damage to healthy cells anywhere in the body. Chemicals that enter the brain can impact it in a way to raise aggression while simultaneously causing other learning disorders. It is no wonder that childhood learning disorders are on the rise when babies enter the world with nearly 300 different chemicals that have been measured in their cord blood. The umbilical cord is attached to their body and is how they receive nutrients from the mother, and chemicals into their growing body and brain.

Another way chemicals effect the mind is when one consumes alcohol, drugs or other intoxicants. These intoxicants are designed to release endorphins in the brain causing a type of high, but we know that alcohol destroys nerve endings called dendrites which are responsible for allowing connections to happen from one neuron to the next. Destroying these neurons can increase one's risk of dementia. Medications, street drugs and even cooked oil plaques can all damage nerve endings causing them to die, misfire and prevent connections from happening. A misfiring physical brain can negatively impact your mind taking you out of mindfulness, awareness, and logical smart thinking. You can lose control of your mind and make mindless decisions such as driving a car or riding a bike while intoxicated, walking in traffic, or having unprotected sex for example. Sometimes this intoxicated mindlessness impacts your emotions causing emotional toxicity such as anger, rage, jealousy, depression, and apathy. These emotions can impact your mind again causing it to go into high reactivity mode and you could make mindless choices such as a decision to fight someone or harm someone or harm yourself. You can see how all of the aspects of our human being are interconnected. Feed your mind healthy food including lots of healthy raw fat to protect the neurological connections in the brain. My book, *Panacea,* focuses on the interconnectedness of the different aspects of who we are as a human being and dives much deeper into the topic of uncovering the toxins in all of the aspects of who we are.

Pharmaceuticals/Vaccinations
Pharmaceuticals are mostly synthetic chemicals that have been created to treat symptoms. There is a time and place for pharmaceuticals and if needed, you can bet that if I am ever in a situation where they are necessary, I will take them and be very grateful for

them. However, because they are chemicals, medications are toxins to the body. Aspirin for example, is designed to deaden nerve endings, masking pain. Deadening a nerve ending does not treat the underlying cause, and the impact it has on deadening the nerve has to have some residual trauma on that nerve contributing to neurological disorders.

Medications may serve a temporary purpose, but one has to get to the cause of the illness, and getting to the root cause is rarely addressed. Usually, patients are put on medications to stop the symptoms and they stay on them for long periods of time or indefinitely. We now know that the root cause of ailments is from toxicity and deficiencies.

Vaccinations are loaded with chemicals. Before choosing to vaccinate please check the CDC website for the complete list of chemicals that are in every vaccination so you are educated on exactly what you are injecting into your baby or child. Once you have the list of chemicals, my suggestion is to Google the words "toxicity of" and then add the name of the chemical in the vaccine to learn exactly what you are exposing your child's brain and body to before you make your decision.

Your blood makes a complete circle around your body approximately every minute, so one minute after a vaccination has been given, these chemicals have passed through the brain and all the organs and the entire body. One minute later, they have passed through again, one minute later they have passed through again... Each time they circulate around the body, the chemicals can damage healthy cells in their path.

I am not here to tell you that you should or should not vaccinate as that is a personal decision that is up to you. Some parents don't want their child to go through such intense bacterial or viral detoxifications so they try to prevent them with vaccines which are designed to stop the detoxification process from happening. Other parents don't want to risk putting these chemicals in their child's body, so they don't vaccinate or pick and choose the ones they want. Either way, adding fresh raw fat to the child's diet puts fat into their bloodstream protecting the brain and body of the child.

The child should be getting consistent healthy raw fat in their diet every day to protect them from daily environmental exposure. However, when injections such as vaccinations are to happen, load them up on the healthy fat a few days before and for at least a week afterwards. The fat will help protect them from the chemicals in the vaccine and will also help carry these chemicals out of the body, but they must also exercise. We don't want the fat to store in the body with the toxins in it, we want it moved out.

In summary, if you DO vaccinate, the fat acts as protection from the toxins holding the chemicals as they travel though the body. If you DO NOT vaccinate, the fat helps grab toxins and debris currently already in the body to pull them out, leaving less of a need for a viral or bacterial detox. I will address this further in the section about raw foods.

Food Toxins:

Now I am going to dive into how food can either heal or harm you. Literally every bite of food you put into your body either heals or harms every cell of your body. Following one basic rule can significantly increase your health.

The closer the food is to its original true nature, the healthier it is for you.

We have always known that cooking food destroys nutrients at some level. Science has also shown us that cooking food changes the chemistry of the food producing actual mutagens and carcinogens. Studies conducted by the National Institute of Health concluded that for nearly every food category, the higher the temperatures and the longer food is cooked, the more caustic properties are created in the food, then you put these food toxins into your body. In addition, I told you how our exposure to chemicals damages and sometimes completely destroys healthy cells in our body creating cell corpses, and how our body sees these dead cells as a form of toxins to be removed. The same thing happens in food. Cooked food was once alive, made up of healthy cells, whether plant or animal cells, they were alive. When you cook the food, you destroy these living cells. Now, when you put these dead food cells into your body you are adding additional dead cells for the body to have to remove. You are adding to the Toxic Body Load.

If you heat up a hot pan and place your hand down on the pan, what would happen? Your healthy skin cells would be instantly destroyed...killed. Your body would move fluids and nutrients to the area to help generate new cells while getting rid of the old dead skin cells, detoxing them from your body. The higher the temperature of the pan and the longer you hold your hand on it, the more damage is done. The same thing happens with food. The higher the temperature the food is cooked at, and the longer you cook it, the more damage is done to the cells of the food, destroying the cells and destroying nutrients, while simultaneously creating toxins.

HOW HEAT AFFECTS DIFFERENT FOOD GROUPS

Destroying nutrients in food affects how that food assimilates in the body and causes toxic residues that store there.

Fats
Read this one carefully. Heart disease is currently the number one killer in the world and heated fats are one of the primary reasons. Heated fats, especially heated nut and seed oils (which many call vegetable oils), are one of the worst things we can put into our body and these heated oils are in everything. This is because numerous studies show that heating fats over 96° F produce lipid peroxides which are known carcinogens. In addition, when fats are heated, it changes their chemistry, causing them to dry out and harden. These cooked oils, which we call plaque, harden throughout the body such as in the arteries, lymphatic system, nerve endings, in the nerves in the brain, and in the prostate. Any part of the body that has some toxic build-up in it, has a very high chance of having these cooked oils which have hardened and stored there. Cooked fats also cause osteoporosis and brittle bones as proven by the works of Dr. Frances Pottenger. Heart disease, lymphoma, enlarged prostate, MS, ALS, Parkinson's, and dementia have all increased exponentially since the processing and cooking of fats, and especially nut and seed oils. They are one of the

primary factors in the cause of these diseases. Detoxing them from the body can be challenging because this hardened plaque can be difficult to dissolve, but if you stick with it and eat the right foods to assist in this cleansing process, you can remove them from the body over time.

You may be eating cooked fats that you don't even know about. All dairy sold in mainstream stores in our country is pasteurized (cooked). There are only a few states in the country that have approved the sale of "raw" unpasteurized dairy and most are sold in natural grocery stores. Pasteurized dairy reaches temperatures of 145° F - 212° F and the pasteurization process destroys nutrients and essential enzymes. When enzymes are destroyed in the milk this affects the digestibility of the dairy. Many people that believe they have a dairy intolerance do not actually have one but are intolerant to the pasteurized dairy because of its void of digestive enzymes due to heating. Some people may also have an intolerance to the synthetic vitamins that are added as these are man-made chemicals.

In addition, many nut and seed oils that you buy from the grocery store have already been heated to very high temperatures before being bottled and/or may have toxic chemical residues in them from the oil extraction process. There are two primary ways of making edible nut and seed oils. The first is through mechanical pressing and the second way is through solvent extraction.

There is a huge variance in the different types of mechanical presses. Expeller pressing starts out with nutrient rich, healthy, life giving seeds that are mechanically cleaned and hulled and sometimes mashed. They are then cooked for up to two hours in various temperatures averaging around 248° F. The cooked seeds are then pressed in an expeller press that creates additional heat, through friction, of up to 203° F. The result is a mechanically pressed oil that can be labeled "unrefined". There are also other mechanical presses that extract oils but are rarely used because the oil output is much lower.

The second method of removing oil from seed is by solvent extraction. Seeds are ground into meal and mixed with a solvent such as hexane or heptane, both volatile chemicals derived from petroleum. The oil and solvent mixture are then separated from the seed and the solvent is evaporated from the oil at temperatures around 302° F. This widely used method produces the highest oil yields and can leave residual toxic solvents in the oils, so if the company is focused only on cost this is most likely the way they extract their oils. The leftover meal cake with the solvents in it is sold as animal feed. This solvent extraction method does not take into consideration the harmful long-term effects of the people (and animals) consuming the oil. Unfortunately, those most affected are the poor who cannot afford the more expensive hand pressed oils.

Some oils sold under the label as "unrefined" are mixtures of expeller pressed and solvent extracted. Refined oils are commonly taken through even more steps such as degumming, bleaching, and deodorizing. Though it may be hard to believe, the term "cold pressed" that is seen on so many labels truly means nothing, as there are no regulations and anyone can put this label on their oil. Most expeller pressed oils are labeled this way and frequently reach high temperatures.

Not only are the oils heated, but so are some nuts. Packaged "raw almonds" are not raw but are either steam pasteurized or fumigated with the chemical propylene oxide, a highly poisonous chemical that the CDC website reports as a mutagenic chemical that causes cancer. It is an actual law in the United States that almonds must be pasteurized to kill bacteria that may be on the almonds due to two deaths that were blamed on raw almonds. If the deaths were caused by bacteria on the almonds, millions of people would have died over the years from eating almonds. This is completely illogical. The pasteurization and fumigation of the almonds with a caustic chemical will actually contribute to more deaths in the long run than the bacteria causing a massive detoxification of two individuals who were full of poisons. If you pull their medical charts, I am certain you would find the truth; possibly dehydration from not getting enough fluids, possibly a reaction to a medication that was given for the detoxification, or possibly a reaction to an antibiotic that shut the kidneys down, or a toxic body detoxing too quickly without rebuilding new healthy cells at the same time. Could be any number of reactions to poisons, but bacteria are blamed because of our misinformation. Once again, the intention was good, but based on false information to start with.

Heart disease and other degenerative diseases have been on the rise at an astounding rate since people have transitioned from using raw butter and raw animal fat to cook with, to vegetable oils which are so prevalent today. These heated oils are one of our biggest killers. We are told not to eat saturated fats because they cause disease, and they do...... when they are cooked. Raw saturated fats do not harden and cause disease, and are in fact extremely healthy and important for a healthy diet. I am not against nut and seed oils and they too can be extremely healthful and are an important part of a healthy diet when truly raw and unheated, but because of the oil extraction process one must find a clean source. Of course you want to cut out hydrogenated oils immediately. Not only does the hydrogenation process change the natural chemistry of the oil, it also leaves residual caustic compounds from the heavy metals and chemicals used during the process.

Carbohydrates
Cooked carbohydrates such as grains and potatoes produce mutagens that store in the body. The NRC publication, "Diet, Nutrition and Cancer", reported that "the frying of potatoes and the toasting of bread result in the formation of mutagenic activity". A study at Columbia University showed how cooking carbohydrates such as breads, crackers, pasta, cakes, cookies and other products from grains, produced something called Advanced Glycation End Products or glycotoxins. 70% of these toxins store in a healthy person and 90% store in an unhealthy person.

Stockholm University showed that cooking carbohydrates like French fries, potato chips, cakes, and bread, produce acrylamides that are known carcinogens as well as neurotoxins. The British Foods Standard confirmed the study, adding that acrylamides cause gene mutations leading to cancers including: breast, uterine and scrotum. California has this toxin listed on its Prop 65 warning which notifies patrons of food establishments about significant chemicals in their business that cause cancer, neurological damage, birth defects, or reproductive harm. Coffee shops must display this sign due to the fact that roasted coffee has the known carcinogen acrylamides in it due to the heating process that creates the toxin. Only coffee made with unroasted green beans would not contain these caustic compounds. Put in the words: California prop 65 list of chemicals to get the latest list.

It is a good reference for anyone to have, not just Californians.

Animal Protein
Cooking animal protein such as steak, chicken, fish, and pork, changes the chemical makeup of that animal protein and produces carcinogens called heterocyclic amines (or HCAs). The longer muscle meat is cooked and the higher the temperatures of cooking, the higher the rate of toxic HCA's. Scientists have discovered that HCA's have powerful mutagenic activity. One of the interesting findings is that the less fat on the meat, the higher the rate of HCAs. This means that those eating a well-done grilled chicken breast, having been cooked on a very high heat, are getting more HCA's in their food than those eating a rare fatty burger. We also know that saturated fats offer a level of protection and the fat on the burger protects the meat from the HCA impact. It is kind of like how the fatty myelin sheath in the brain protects the nerve cells. When that fat is destroyed by toxins then the toxins can get to the nerve cells. This is the same concept of saturated fats protecting the muscle meat from HCA's. All cooked animal protein however,

has some level of HCAs. Again, the higher the temperature and the longer it is cooked the more HCA's are produced, whereas all raw unheated animal protein contains absolutely no HCAs at all.

The National Research Council, when studying diet as it relates to cancer found that cooking beef stock in temperatures as low as 154°F (less than boiling point), frying fish and broiling hamburgers, all produced mutagens. Studies also show that high temperature dry heat such as grilling, and broiling produce the highest levels. We live in such a bacteria, viral and parasite phobic culture that we are doing everything we can to destroy them; and in the process, destroy not only the microbes that were designed to save us, but also the life giving nutrients in our food, while simultaneously creating toxic substances that store in the body.

Fruits/Vegetables
The cooking of fruits and vegetables destroys vital nutrients. Every cell in our body depends on nutrients for survival. The slightest destruction to these nutrients can affect digestion and absorption in the body. Before man started duplicating fire to use for his own personal gains, we were originally designed to eat food uncooked. Over time, some humans have developed an enzyme mutation to allow the body to digest and assimilate cooked and processed foods, including cooked and processed fruits and vegetables. However, many people still do not have this enzyme mutation and the residues of cooked and processed fruits and vegetables remain in their body causing health problems. This is one of the reasons why juicing is so healthful for you as the produce used to make fresh juice is raw and the juice from fresh

pressed fruits and vegetables can immediately assimilate right into your cells when you drink it.

The latest buzz word today is "phytonutrients". These are found in the skins of mostly fruits and vegetables and are in fact what give them their pigmentation (or color). Studies are showing their beneficial factors in enhancing the immune system and possibly preventing some forms of cancer. When scientists discover a certain phytonutrient from a particular food, it is assumed that all forms of that food contain the beneficial phytonutrient...this is not the case. Grapes for example, contain Flavonoids that carry many health benefits. It does not mean that grape juice also carries those same benefits as it is pasteurized at temperatures of over 140°F. The only way to get the full nutrition value of the grape is to eat the raw grapes themselves in whole or pressed juice form. There are some fruits and vegetables that when cooked increase certain nutrients. Tomatoes are a perfect example. When tomatoes are heated the lycopene levels increase, but what happens to the levels of the other nutrients? Additionally, if you grill your fruits and vegetables as is very popular in the summer months, you produce additional carcinogenic properties from the char grilling.

With all foods, the higher the heat and the longer it is cooked, the more toxic it is for the body.

DEFICIENCIES

Deficiencies are the second cause of disease. If toxins destroy healthy cells causing cellular death, so do deficiencies. When healthy cells do not get the nutrients they need to survive, they weaken and/or die off. When this happens, we are once again creating cellular debris and cell corpses. The human body looks at cellular debris the same as it does toxins and does what it has to do to cleanse them out of the body. It brings fluids to the area to try to flush them out the most efficient route. Think about how when you were a kid and you got a splinter in your hand. The area around the splinter would swell up as your body was trying to push it out with fluid. The same thing happens inside the body when toxins are present. The body sends fluids to the area of the poisons to flush them out and they exit through any possible orifice of the body. Deficiencies occur due to our poor diets. Our bodies and body parts are starving for nutrients, but instead of real whole live foods, we feed it highly processed, over cooked death.

The combination of toxemia through various sources, and nutritional deficiencies, are what create the toxic host. They can also contribute to DNA mutations inside of us and we pass those mutated DNA to our children. Our children continue to eat the cooked and processed foods that leave toxic residues in their bodies and are exposed to more and more environmental poisons, and their DNA mutates further, and they pass these genes to their children. Yes, some mutations can be beneficial as that is how we have evolved over the years to adapt to our environment, but DNA mutations caused by caustic poisons damage parts of the body that negatively affect our health and life and become part of our genetic make-up that we pass to generations to come.

What are we creating? Every year there are more birth defects, a higher percentage of childhood neurological disorders such as Autism and ADD, increases in heart disease, cancer, chronic illness, pain, etc. Cellular destruction and mutations are not always obvious at first. The first one or two generations may not physically see or feel it, but eventually someone down the genetic line will have to live with the consequences. It is no wonder that children are born today with devastating diseases and that adults are plagued with chronic conditions developing so early in life. We have some of the best physicians in the world and spend more money on the health industry than any other country and yet the percentage of people suffering disease is not decreasing..... its increasing every year.

Our current generation is a perfect example of how generational lung poisoning can occur. Great grandparents and grandparents who smoked and destroyed the genes of their lungs passed those genes to their children who may have also smoked doing even more harm to their lung genetics. Even if there was a generation who chose not to smoke, it is still possible that their children can be born with chronic respiratory conditions such as asthma as is happening today. The toxins are passed on to the innocent. The same thing is happening to babies of mothers who are exposed to lead in drinking water, environmental radiation, household chemicals and cleaning products, pesticides and herbicides, skin care products, etc. These micro poisonings are damaging your insides without you knowing it and you will pass these poisons and damaged organs to your unborn children.

The medical community does nothing to address this issue of toxicity causing the illnesses we have today. Its only focus is on treating symptoms through drug therapy without enough research on the causes of disease... the "why". This is what physicians are trained to do in medical school. Don't get me wrong, I have great appreciation for physicians, but the bulk of medicine is managing chronic symptoms with drug therapy and is based on this germ theory that the microbes as the cause, which is absolutely not the case. There are times that drug therapy needs to be used to get a condition under control or to relieve pain until we can slowly detoxify the body. I am also not saying we need to live our lives in dirty conditions. There are some places that we want kept completely sterile such as hospitals, medical facilities, and nail salons. These are the places where we want the cleaning agents to be used. There are natural cleaning agents on the market today that are even more effective than chemicals and yet safe enough to spray in the mouth.

One of the original founders of the Food and Drug Administration, Dr. Harvey Wiley, spoke of how the ingredients of cold and cough remedies all contain poisons that relieve conditions by suppressing the "detoxification process", thereby pushing all of the toxins trying to get out back into the body and adding additional drug poisons. Dr. Wiley was later forced from his position at the FDA because of his great knowledge on the natural healing effects of the body and the poisonous effects of pharmaceuticals.

The amazing thing is that the body will do its job if given the right tools. Its job is detoxification and healing, and the tools are natural bacteria, viruses, parasites and molds, healthy raw foods, exercise, rest and a positive mental attitude.

"Thy food shall be thy remedy"- Hippocrates

STATISTICS

Unfortunately, the chances are that you will actually be one of these statistics unless you wake-up and make the changes you need to make today. The United States spends more on pharmaceuticals and healthcare than any other country in the world and yet we have some of the highest rates of chronic illness.

• Approximately 50% of all Americans will die of Heart Disease at some point in their life.

• 90% of Americans 55 or older are at risk of hypertension or heart disease.

• 1.7 M new cases of cancer are expected to be diagnosed in 2018 (excluding skin cancers) and 609,000 people will die from cancer.

• In 2017, 30.3M American adults had Diabetes. It has now reached epidemic proportions and is the 7th leading cause of death.

• An estimated 90% of Americans who are pre-diabetic do not even know it.

• Nearly 6M Americans of all ages have Alzheimer's disease as of 2017. According to the Alzheimer's Association, that number is expected to triple to nearly 18M by 2050.

• In the United States, 58M Americans are overweight, 40M are obese and 3M are morbidly obese.

• In less than 15 years, 50% of all adults in the U.S will be obese.

• According to the CDC in 2014, the prevalence of Autism in US children   increased by 119.4% from 1 in 150 kids in 2000 to the current rate of 1 in 68.

• 1.5M Americans have an Autism spectrum disorder. Autism is the fastest growing developmental disease.

THE SECRET TO HEATH:
DETOX – REBUILD – REPEAT

There is a lot of talk about detoxification and cleanses but also much confusion. Seems everyone is on a cleanse these days. I saw a box of herbs at the checkout stand that were labeled "liver detox". Can herbs actually detox a liver? Let's dive into the subject and demystify detoxification. Detoxification means to remove toxic substances... De = remove + tox = toxins. This is exactly what we want to do... remove the poisons that we have been exposed to, including dead cells and debris, from the body. There are many products out there that claim to "detox" the body, but exactly how do they do this? I am going to talk about natural ways to clean out the garbage and how you are already helping it along with some foods you eat today.

The liver and kidneys are the two organs we most associate with the cleansing of the body as they act like filters for the poisons. But because we have more poisons coming into our body and we are creating more dead cells than our body is eliminating, we must find a way to assist the detoxification process.

All toxins have a positive ionic charge to them, some a stronger charge than others. Interesting to also know that all cooked foods also have a positive ionic charge to them because we create the toxins from the cooking process. So if you put something in the body that has a negative ionic charge to it, it bonds with the positive ions of the poisons and detoxifies the body. This is called chelation. <u>All foods in their raw unheated form have a negative ionic charge to them and detox the body</u>. That means raw unpasteurized dairy, raw eggs, raw nut and seed oils, raw fruits and vegetables and their juices, raw fish, raw meat, and raw honey. When a newborn baby nurses, they are getting fresh raw milk from mom and are actually detoxing. This is one of the reasons why babies who nurse from a healthy mother rarely become ill or go through detoxification, because the raw mother's milk puts them through little continual mini detoxes. The longer a mother nurses the better for a baby.

The Juice Cleanse
What about juice cleanses, herbal cleanses, and colon hydrotherapy? Fresh pressed juices are packed with nutrients and I call them vitamins in a bottle because your body does not have to breakdown the cellulose to utilize the nutrients and send them right into your cells. If the juice is made with fresh raw vegetables and fruits, then this juice has a negative ionic charge to it and yes, it is actually cleansing toxins from your body. If however, the juice is made with pasteurized or heated vegetables and fruits, as are from the traditional jars of juice on the shelves, the ionic charge is now positive and detoxification is not occurring in the body. In addition, the heating process has destroyed many of the vital nutrients in the juice and in this case, you are not only not detoxing, but actually adding residues to the body from the cooking process with the level of residues related to the cooking method.

Being on a strict juice cleanse is cause for concern if done for an extended period of time because of the lack of fat and protein consumed. When consuming fresh pressed juice, the negative ionic charge can free stored toxins and help move them out of the body, but if there is not proper healthy raw fat in the body and blood at the time of this detoxification process, these toxins can either do additional damage or re-store somewhere else on their journey out. For example, if a heavy metal such as lead were released from the brain and into the body from a juice cleanse, and it gets dumped into the intestinal system for removal, unless there is fat in the intestinal system to protect the G.I. tract, that lead could do severe damage, or re-store in the intestines or colon on its way out of the body. Gastrointestinal disorders increase every year due to poisons doing damage trying to get out of the body. Healthy raw fat is essential to protection. If you are on a fresh pressed raw juice cleanse, you MUST have healthy raw fats as part of that cleanse. Mix fresh raw coconut cream, or raw dairy into your juice or have some between juices to get the fat into your body. Another option is to blend fresh avocado into your green juices for added fat protection.

If one does not have the vegetarian gene, as is the bulk of the population in the United States, the lack of protein when on a strict juice cleanse can be another concern. When the body is going through a detoxification, it is crucial that it also be rebuilding at the same time. Protein is one of the most important building blocks to regenerating new healthy cells. Visualize the negative ionic charge of the juice pulling toxins and cellular corpses out, and out, and out. This is great to be moving all of this debris out of the body, but for many people who have a lot of accumulated debris, it can be too much and can actually weaken them very quickly.

Imagine an old home that was built with wood 2 x 4's and asbestos panels. Someone comes in and says this asbestos is toxic and we need to get it out and they pull out all of the panels leaving only the old wood supports. The toxic stuff is gone, but the structure as a whole has been weakened. Even though the asbestos was toxic, its panels gave the house some strength in structure and now that it is gone. The home overall is weaker until the new panels are put up made with healthy materials. This is like the body. If you just keep detoxing and detoxing and detoxing without rebuilding at the same time, you can weaken the body.

I have a client who went on a very strict vegan raw diet. He became very weak, had brain fog, and some real health challenges. Although he has not yet been tested for the vegetarian gene, we are pretty certain he does not have it. If he had been on a balanced detox plan where he could have been rebuilding new healthy cells with raw or very rare animal protein, he most likely could have kept doing the juices, but instead he stopped the whole thing and went back to his old ways of eating toxic foods. You MUST rebuild while detoxing. This is why if you do not have the vegetarian gene, you must have raw or rare animal protein in your diet.

The Herbal Detox
Herbs are frequently marketed as detox remedies but let's look at this carefully. Herbs are not actually removing toxins from the body unless they are dried at very low temperatures preserving the negative ionic charge, but they do support organs in functioning

better by providing nutrients that support the organs. When the organ functions better, it can move poisons out of the body much more efficiently, allowing for an increase in toxin removal.

However, if the herbs are fresh, they can be put into a juicer and juiced in which they will not only support the liver in working better, but the negative ionic charge of the fresh juiced herbs will detox poisons. I am a big fan of juicing herbs for this reason.

Colon Hydrotherapy
There is a time and place for colon hydrotherapy (or colonics), but in my opinion they are being used much too frequently and they are destroying the G.I. tract. Colonics are promoted as being a cure-all for the gut as the water injected into the colon through the rectum flushes out the poisons stored there. This may actually happen, but just like how chemotherapy destroys the good cells along with the bad cells, so do colonics remove all of the intestinal bacteria along with the toxins. G.I. bacteria is used to continue to breakdown food in addition to cellular debris and poisons, and these bacteria can take years to accumulate and get into balance. With one flush of the colon, you can wipe out years of work. In my opinion, it is better to flush out toxins in the colon from the top down. Eating foods that detoxify the body along with plenty of healthy raw fat will pick up the poisons in the colon as they move through, and the raw fat and raw protein will rebuild the new healthy cells healing instead of harming.

MEAT EATERS VS VEGETARIANS

There is no doubt in my mind after researching this subject that humans were naturally very much meat eaters from the beginning, as Anthropological evidence supports this. Evolution has happened in various parts of the world where vegetarian diets have been adopted out of necessity or choice, which has created a genetic mutation to allow for this, but as far as we can tell, today the majority of the world's population still needs some level of animal protein for survival.

About four million years ago, the first humans (the Australopithecines) ate a large amount of small animals and were scavengers of the remains of large animals. They ate some plant foods, but their main source of nutrition was animal protein. Man evolved into Peking and Java man, Neanderthal man and Cro-Magnon man. As this evolution took place, man increased his ability to hunt and was able to capture and eat wild game. Although man was omnivorous, from the very beginning his diet relied heavily on meats.

It is thought that agriculture began about ten thousand years ago when wild game started to become exhausted. However, crops were not grown for eating. They were grown to begin raising domesticated animals for their meat. A bone found from a woman dating 5735-5630 BC, in the United Kingdom, proved "the woman's diet was virtually as meat-rich as that of a carnivorous wild animal". Near her thigh bone was found the bones of aurochs, deer and otter.

The Neolithic period, 4100-2000BC, has been associated as the period that farming began. Stable isotopes have been used to measure the amounts of bone protein in the bone of Britain's Neolithic man. The levels were sometimes higher than that of a carnivorous animal. These so called 'first farmers' were eating large amounts of meats, including animal products such as dairy.

As wild game became scarce, man settled down to raise domesticated animals for meat. There began the formation of organized religion. As this occurred, some religious groups gradually adopted "no meat" beliefs. Anthropologist Marvin Harris points out that Hindus were meat eaters before they converted to vegetarianism. And, the Dali Lama began eating animal meats after being advised by his physicians that he needed this to improve his health.

There is evidence that no ancient culture around the world has ever been totally vegetarian. Each has always had some sort of animal meat in its diet. Doctors Weston Price and Francis Pottenger traveled around the world in the 1930's and during this time, they could not find one long-lived society on our planet that was primarily vegetarian. On the contrary, there are numerous cultures that lived almost exclusively on meats and meat fats such as the Eskimos that were studied by anthropologist Vilhjalmur Stefansson, as well as many tribes in Africa.

In addition to this Anthropological evidence, we can take a look at how the intestines are designed in man versus animals that consume primarily vegetation. Nutritional consultant and primal diet creator, Aajonus Vonderplanitz, describes how humans are not designed to digest raw whole vegetables and grains. He sites our intestines being 2 1⁄2 times shorter than herbivores and the fact that we have only one stomach as opposed to the 2-4 stomachs of an herbivore as evidence. "Herbivores have nearly 60,000 times more enzymes than humans to disassemble plant fiber to obtain the fat and proteins from vegetation and grain. Vegetable fiber passes through an herbivores digestive system in about 48 hours. In humans, it passes through in 24 hours with only 1/3-1/2 of the cellulose digested, leaving most of the protein and fat undigested. Basically, we don't digest raw whole vegetables and grain very well. We cannot utilize that which we cannot digest", says Vonderplanitz.

THE FOOD GRADIENT:
FROM WELL DONE TO RAW

Truly nutritional foods are in their purest form. The cultures that consume the most processed foods have the highest rates of chronic and degenerative disease. The closer a food is to its true nature, the healthier it is, and each level of processing increases its toxicity level. The next time you walk through a grocery store, really look at what is "alive" in the store....not much. Only "live" foods can be found around the perimeter of the store and include meat, dairy, fruits, vegetables, nuts and seeds, and many of these pure whole foods have been altered to some degree. Some meats have been raised with medications and hormones, had chemicals put on them during slaughter, and some have additional chemicals added after processing to preserve their freshness. You may believe that when you buy a piece of meat from your local grocer that it is fresh meat with nothing added, but this may not be true. This statement below was taken directly from the USDA website.

Natural Products

All raw single ingredient meat and poultry qualify as "natural." However, certain products labeled as natural may also contain a flavoring solution provided the solution contains ingredients that are minimally processed and not artificial; e.g., natural flavoring. The amount of solution added to products bearing natural claims is not limited. All products claiming to be *natural* should be accompanied by a brief statement which explains what is meant by the term "natural." Source: USDA website.

This means a grocery store could legally advertise their meat as "natural" and it could have so-called "natural flavoring" added. The FDA considers 3000 chemical food additives to be labeled as "natural flavors". This is not only for packaged meats, but every processed food on the shelf as well. In addition, up to 70% of grocery store meats have been gassed with carbon monoxide to keep the meat bright red and prevent it from turning brown as it would do naturally. Most packaged meats have had gas added to it as it lasts longer on the shelves. I buy my meats from the meat counter at Wholefoods. I was told they do not gas their meat or meat case, but instead they are on a tight order schedule, ordering only minimal meats that will sell within 3 days. When the meat begins to turn brown, it is pulled and discarded. Add natural flavors and carbon monoxide to your list of chemicals doing damage to the healthy cells in your body. This does not mean you should stop eating meat. There is a gradient. Antibiotic and hormone free meat is better than meat with these medications. Meat without natural flavorings are better than those that have them. Meats that have not been gassed are better than those that have been gassed.

As a side note: this procedure of discarding meat that has turned brown is unfortunate as this brown meat is in the beginning stages of growing good bacteria that if eaten, can breakdown toxins in the body and brain to help reverse cancer, depression and other health conditions. Indigenous cultures around the world would age meat and eat it for detoxification purposes. We now understand the gut brain connection and many people who suffer from depression eat aged meats to support their mental health.

Dairy products that were once delivered fresh to homes straight from the farm are now pasteurized and homogenized removing the natural enzymes, destroying nutrients, and adding synthetic/chemical vitamins. Even dairy is not really alive any longer unless you are one of the very fortunate to live in a state that has legalized raw unpasteurized dairy. As you are beginning to see, the techniques that are practiced are designed with good intent, to keep the food products from growing bacteria so they will last longer on the shelves, but what is happening is the exact opposite. These chemicals are poisoning our body and now we are not getting the natural bacteria our body needs to breakdown poisons in the body. We are doing the opposite of what our body really needs.

Fruits and vegetables are grown in mineral depleted soil, and sprayed with pesticides, herbicides and fungicides. When produce with these toxins are cooked, the degree of poison is exacerbated as the heating process usually makes a toxin more toxic. Look for organic and non-GMO produce. In addition, nuts and seeds are not being pasteurized.

The vast majority of foods found in grocery stores, even natural food stores, are dead, processed foods. Nearly everything in the center sections of the store are dead foods, and frequently the fresh live foods we buy, we then cook to death. This does not mean you can never eat processed foods. Again, this is about increased awareness. When picking a processed food, look for the least processed. Baking is better than frying, and dehydrating at low temps is better than baking. There is a gradient.

Cooking kills...the food and eventually us. Life begets life!

When I am speaking of eating raw unheated foods, I am not talking about a life of salads, sprouting and dehydrating nuts and seeds. Modern science shows us that the majority of humans around the world should not be on a strict vegan diet as it could be very detrimental to their health, unless they have the vegetarian allele (vegetarian gene). As referenced earlier, a study at Cornell University showed that only 18% of Americans actually have the vegetarian gene and can survive on a vegetarian diet alone. Individuals from South Africa and South Asia had up to a 55% rate of this vegetarian genetic mutation, hinting that if you have these roots in your heritage, you may have this gene.

My research shows that most of us are still genetically designed to be meat eaters and that our bodies need animal proteins to live with radiant health. Most people use protein powders to supplement their diets when the egg is the perfect protein and are what all protein powders are designed to simulate. That is why Rocky ate raw eggs all the time.

When eating raw foods, your body is constantly going through a detoxification process. This is because toxins have a positive ionic charge. Cooked food also has a positive ionic charge. The more it is cooked and the higher the temperatures, the higher the positive charge. All food in its unheated raw form has a negative ionic charge to it including raw unpasteurized dairy (milk, cream, and butter), raw eggs, raw meat of any kind, raw fruits and vegetables and their raw juices, raw nuts and seeds and their oils. When you eat anything raw, the negative ionic charge of the raw food binds with the positive ionic charge of toxins carrying them out of the body.

When you eat an apple, you are detoxing. When you eat a salad you are detoxing. When you eat sushi you are detoxing (unless you are eating Americanized cooked sushi). When you eat ceviche' from Mexican restaurants you are detoxing. When you eat carpaccio from Italian restaurants you are detoxing. When you eat Poke' you are detoxing. When you eat kibbe from a middle eastern restaurant you are detoxing. Anything uncooked has a negative ionic charge to it. Once again, the longer food is cooked and the higher the temperatures, the less negative charge it has to it, the more positive charge is created, and the more chemical reactions happen causing caustic compounds.

In addition to unheated foods detoxifying your body, they also help rebuild and repair the body and help regenerate new healthy cells.

Raw Fats:
Raw fats are one of the most crucial foods required for radiant health. Yes, I just said fat! Raw fats come in the form of raw eggs, raw unpasteurized dairy (milk, cream, kefir, cheese and butter), fresh raw coconut

cream or truly unheated coconut oil, raw avocado, raw nuts and seeds and their unheated oils. The importance of healthy raw fat is vital to protect the body from poisons, lubricate arteries, the G.I tract, lymph, and nerves, and it fuels the body. Repeated studies have shown that diets low in fat have been associated with depression, cancer, psychological disorders, fatigue, suicide and violence. Harvard University proved that the modern day, low fat diet has caused an alarming increase in degenerative disorders.

I have a personal story related to this subject in which my uncle, who was a brilliant engineer for one of the major car companies, was put on a low to no-fat diet by his physician for "health reasons" when he retired. Within 2 years he developed Parkinson's disease, post-polio syndrome, and paranoia...all are neurological disorders exacerbated from the lack of fat. The brain is over 60% fat and cholesterol and the myelin that covers neurons in the brain are 70% fat. The reason the brain is so high in fat is for protective reasons because the neurological connections are so essential to our survival. If the brain and mind are not working together it severely impacts the life of the individual. We desperately need beneficial raw fats and cholesterol to maintain healthy brain and nervous system function. If you have any kind of neurological issues, load up on raw fat to soothe damaged nerves.

Raw fats also protect the body from toxins by binding with them so the toxins can be removed safely. When I had mercury amalgams removed from my mouth I began experiencing a burning in my esophagus and stomach. It was excruciatingly painful. I realized the toxic mercury was dumping into my G.I. tract for removal from my body, but because I did not have enough fats in my diet at the time, the mercury was burning my G.I. tract on its way out of my body causing the discomfort. I immediately started drinking a mixture of raw eggs, raw cream and raw unheated honey. The pain dissipated within 10 minutes. I continued to drink this mixture to coat and protect my esophagus for two weeks. I needed the mucus layer for protection against the toxic metals.

Raw dairy has been shown to be one of the most beneficial and healing foods around. Raw milk was used by ancient physicians Hippocrates and Galen to cure diseases, by Dr. J.E. Crewe of the Mayo Foundation to cure TB, high blood pressure, prostate disease, diabetes, kidney disease, chronic fatigue and obesity. The theory as to why raw milk is so successful in treatments is because raw dairy contains natural microbes that assist in breaking down toxins and debris, it contains raw fat which can then engulf the toxins and debris carrying them out of the body, and its protein is complete providing all of the amino acids necessary for rebuilding healthy new cells.

Nature gives us an abundance of animals that provide health giving milk: cow, sheep, goats, camels, buffalo, yaks, oxen, antelope, reindeer and zebras for example. The milk can be consumed as-is, or made into kefir or yogurt that is full of good bacteria. The cream from the milk can also be consumed as-is or made into butter. Some of the earliest human artifacts include pots that contain traces of milk residue. In fact, historians believe milk consumption dates back at least 30,000 years with the beginning of civilization.

<u>Raw Meats</u>
When it was found that cooking meats causes mutagens that cause cancer, many thought the solution was to not eat meat at all. However, if you do not have the vegetarian gene, raw meats are crucial to the healing process. They are necessary in regenerating cells in our body. As I described in the section on detoxification, after a bacteria, virus, parasite or mold breaks down degenerative tissue for efficient elimination, it is important to our health that we eat the proper foods to then regenerate new cells in this area. Raw animal meats, especially in combination with a raw fat, will regenerate new cells faster than any other food because all of its amino acids are intact.

When protein is consumed, it breaks down into amino acids. Then, when a certain part of the body needs to repair itself, it uses a very specific amino acid combination that is determined by your personal DNA. Since amino acids are destroyed from heat and cooking, when it is time to do repair work in the body, or let's say to regrow new cells or repair an organ, if the amino acids were destroyed by heat, you will not have the amino acid combination for this repair work.

For example, if you were exposed to some household chemicals that damaged your lungs and kidneys, you need the proper nutrients, including protein (amino acids) to repair those areas. Maybe your DNA says that you need the ABCD amino acid combination to repair your lungs and kidneys, but you eat your animal protein well done and in doing so you have destroyed all of the B and C amino acids. Now when your lungs and kidneys need that entire ABCD combination for repair, it does not have the entire combination because you destroyed the B and C amino acids so repair cannot happen. If you eat your meat cooked medium to rare, maybe you destroy some of the amino acids but not all of them so you may have enough to repair one organ but not the other. On the other hand, if you eat your animal protein unheated and raw, ALL of the amino acids are intact and you have enough for the rebuilding of both organs. Plus, as a bonus, you have not created additional cooking toxins that you are putting into your body. It's a win-win.

This is exactly one of the primary reasons why our hormones get out of balance as we age. We do not have all of the essential amino acids necessary to support the survival and rebuilding of our hormones, so they are deficient in our body.

As I already touched on, all meat is not alike as the source is important. If you have the means to buy organic and 100% grass-fed, that is always the best, but there are gradients of meat quality based on the conditions of how the animals are kept and how they are treated, the level of medications given to the animals, and the quality of food they eat. Processed genetically modified soy and corn are common fillers to animal food and are not healthy for the animal or the person eating the meat of the animal eating the GMO food. Read labels and do your research.

The same way that heating destroys healthy cells in meat, freezing also destroys healthy cells in animal protein. The following was taken from the USDA website describing how the water in meat freezes and the sharp frozen edges poke into the cells of the meat destroying them and leaving the dead cells in the meat. Thus, the healthiest animal product to eat is fresh, previously unfrozen, raw animal protein. If you are going to cook your animal protein, you want to again use fresh not previously frozen and you will be destroying healthy cells upon freezing and then again upon the heating of the protein.

Freezing Meat and Poultry
When meat and poultry are frozen, the water that is a natural component of all meats turns to solid ice crystals. The water expands when it freezes. The sharp-edged crystals push into the surrounding tissue, rupturing the cells. The water that is outside the cell membrane freezes first. As it does, it leeches water from inside the cell membranes. When it thaws, the original balance does not return to normal. The thawed product will have lost some of its natural springiness. The water released during freezing seeps out of the thawing meat and poultry into the package. Source: USDA website.

When stating out eating raw meat, everyone is different. Some people just go for it, and others like to gradually increase the bacterial levels they ingest. Some people marinate meats in sauces made with raw apple cider vinegar and citrus, such as in the recipes I have in the back of this book. The high acidity levels of the cider vinegar and citrus kills the bacteria on the meat. Others like to start with frozen meats so any parasite that may be in the meat is destroyed.

When choosing eggs to eat raw, consider the following. "Pasture eggs" are theoretically the best, followed by "free-range". Pastured means they were actually raised in a pasture where they have lots of room to roam in an open area and ate what chickens are designed to eat.... bugs and vegetation. Contrary to popular belief, "free-range" and "cage-free" does not mean they have any more than 1 – 2 square feet to move. There is much more to it than this, but that is the general rule of thumb when buying store-bought eggs.

The absolute best way to have eggs is to raise them yourself. This way you know exactly what they have been exposed to, what they are eating, and how much room they have to roam. Everything the chicken eats and is exposed to is what you will be eating. Fed them every leftover scrap you have and allow them to eat bugs and worms and give them lots of love. Happy chickens are healthy and nourish your body better than the eggs of stressed chickens. In addition, store-bought eggs have been washed in chemicals by law. Egg shells are porous and absorb these chemicals into the eggs which you then eat. If you cook them, you risk the chemical being altered even more and becoming even more toxic to your body.

If you raise your own chickens, collect the eggs each day and put them in a basket on your counter. The healthiest eggs are non-refrigerated. There is a protective coating on the egg that allows them to remain on the counter unrefrigerated for 2 weeks (although I have had some unwashed unrefrigerated for a month), and 3 months refrigerated. If you have any concern about an egg having too much bacteria in it, just smell it. The human nose can detect bacteria so crack the egg into a cup and smell it. If there is no smell at all, it is good to use. If however you smell any odor, toss it out. A fresh egg has no odor. In my first 16 years of eating raw eggs, I have had probably 3 bad eggs. If you do not raise your eggs, check out neighbor social media postings. I have found eggs raised and fed the way I would in local area. I just tell them how many dozen unwashed unrefrigerated eggs I would like, and they save them for me to pick up.

Raw Fruits & Vegetables
Drink your vegetables whenever possible! Because the Standard American Diet is so void of nutrition, this is a great way to pack in the vitamins, minerals, and nutrients. Fresh-pressed raw green vegetable juices are also important to alkalinize the blood and urine helping keep us in balance. Another purpose for these juices is to hydrate and oxygenate our cells. I tend to push green juices because not only are most people void of the nutrients from green leafy vegetables, many others have sugar issues and need to be cautious with too much juice made from fruits and root vegetables. My green juice is usually a base of celery and cucumber, with either a green leafy vegetable such as parsley or spinach. Then I add other fruits and vegetables for taste such as ginger, lemon, apple and pineapple. I confess drinking green juices are my least favorite thing to consume, but because you are drinking the fresh-pressed juice and not eating the whole vegetable, the juice goes right into your cells without having to breakdown all of the cellulose first to get to the nutrients inside. When I drink it I just think to myself... "this is my medicine". I also add fresh raw unpasteurized milk or cream or some fresh coconut cream to the juice. It gives it that added fat to absorb with the toxins that are being pulled from the body and also gives it a softer taste.

Fruits are also full of high-quality nutrients and should be eaten in their raw form when possible. The amount of fruit each individual can eat may once again be determined by ones genes. One person with pacific island heritage may be able to consume large amounts of fruits while another much less. Someone who has destroyed their pancreas, will most likely not be able to eat as many high sugar fruits as someone with a healthier pancreas. As always, go by how you feel and if there is concern about sugar levels in the blood, eating raw fat such raw unpasteurized dairy, avocado, cheese or fresh raw coconut cream with fruit can slow down the release of sugar into the bloodstream and body.

Of course, consume organic produce whenever possible and supporting your local organic farmer is always a bonus. Not only are conventionally raised fruits and vegetables full of pesticides, herbicides and some are now irradiated, they are very low in minerals due to the depleted soils they are grown in today. As the U.S. demand for organic produce increases, it has had to turn to imports from other countries creating a growing concern about the authenticity of the organics imported. Growing your own garden is the only way to truly know where your produce comes from.

Raw Nuts
Raw nuts can be eaten but be wary that the human body is not designed to digest large amounts of nuts and seeds, causing stomach upset and discomfort. Think about how nuts are found in the wild. It takes quite a long time to remove the shell from just one nut to get to the edible center. If we were to eat them in the wild, we would probably eat only small amounts and very slowly.

Nuts contain enzyme inhibitors such as phytic acid that prevent proper digestion, can cause mineral loss, and can interfere with protein absorption. This is why soaking and sprouting nuts has become so popular today as it deactivates the enzyme inhibitors. There are many small companies making sprouted nuts and seeds that are very healthful.

Raw Honey – the only food that lasts forever!
When I refer to raw honey, I am referring to honey that has come right from the hive without any sort of heat application whatsoever. Raw, unheated honey is in its purest form and has not been subjected to any kind of heat during its processing or packaging, but it is not so easy to find. This is because the majority of beekeepers warm their honey to 100°F or higher to get the honey to flow into the jars.

Raw honey has more than 75 different compounds, is loaded with enzymes, and is being touted as one of today's "superfoods". Enzymes are catalysts for biochemical reactions in the body and are necessary for our bodies to function properly, and since we destroy so many of them when we cook our food, the enzymes in raw honey can help digest even the cooked foods that we eat.

As with all foods, when honey is heated over certain temperatures, the heat destroys its enzymes in addition to the natural insulin-like substances in it. Studies have shown us that on very hot days, the bees work together to fan the hives keeping them at 95°F (35°C), which is the ideal temperature for making honey in the hives. Healthy hives have temperatures that have topped out at about 98°F, but rarely rises above this 98-degree mark. This means when the honey is being packaged for wholesale or retail sale, it should not be labeled "raw honey" if it has reached temperatures above 98°F, but we know that this mislabeling is happening because there are no "raw" labeling regulations. The only way to know definitively that your honey has not been heated is to have bees yourself, which is not as difficult as one might think. There is a beekeeper in Boulder, Colorado that makes a hive called a top-bar hive that can be put on the balcony of an apartment building. If you are interested, contact Corwin Bell at www.BackyardHIve.com. Another option is to go see the beekeeper yourself and ask lots of questions about their process, including the highest temperature reached when packaging.

Eating raw honey throughout the day can reverse diabetes because truly raw unheated honey has natural insulin-like substances which keep the blood-sugar levels level. A beekeeper I work with in Michigan was told by his doctor after having his A1C blood sugar test come back at 4.9, to "Keep doing what you are doing. I don't know if it's all the raw honey you eat or the bee stings but, a 4.9 A1C blood level is excellent." This man is 69 years old and is not a raw foodist, other than some fresh fruits and vegetables that he eats, but the raw honey alone keeps his sugar at healthy levels. When honey is heated over 104°F, it turns into radical sugar that is just as toxic as table sugar in the body. Once again, ask questions and know your sources.

Raw unheated honey is also being rediscovered once again for its medicinal qualities and used by physicians for wound healing. There are now companies that sell sterile pads with raw honey saturated into the pad to be used for wound care and can be purchased at local pharmacies. This is an expensive way to go when you can stick your finger into a jar of raw honey, dab a bit on your wound and cover it with a bandage and it will cost you a few pennies. Plastic surgeons are even getting on the bandwagon suggesting raw honey, raw coconut oil and fresh aloe gel for fast recovery of scars after surgery.

The health benefits of raw honey are not new. It has been used in combination with natural mineral water and lemon for over 5000 years in Ayurvedic medicine for weight loss. Ancient medical scriptures show the benefits of honey include: improved digestion, improved eyesight, soothes a sore throat, gives suppleness to your body, purifies and heals ulcers, gives color to complexion, improves intelligence, cures many types of disease, and heals wounds. Dr. Peter C. Molan, department biological sciences at the University of Waikato, Hamilton, New Zealand, published a report summarizing over 97 different studies on the effects of raw honey. His report is entitled, "Honey as a Dressing for Wounds, Burns and Ulcers: A Brief Review of Clinical Reports and Experimental Studies" sites the following results:

- Infection is rapidly cleared
- Inflammation and swelling quickly reduced
- Odor is reduced
- Sloughing of necrotic tissue is induced
- Healing occurs rapidly with minimal scarring
- Caused no tissue damage
- Promotes the healing process
- Burns heal rapidly without secondary infection
- Sloughs gangrenous tissue

- Increased blood flow in wounds noticed
- Healed ulcers & burns faster than any other local application used before
- Helps skin regenerate, making plastic reconstructive surgery unnecessary
- Reduces edema
- Reduces pain from burns

Other Raw Ingredients

There are other raw ingredients that can be used in recipes when preparing foods. These include raw apple cider vinegar, herbs and spices, raw cacao and raw carob for example. Dried spices can be used but make sure to use a quality brand of organic spices as most all non-organic dried spices have been irradiated.

ADDITIONAL EVIDENCE

Dr Weston Price, a dentist from Cleveland, Ohio, noticed that his patients were developing more and more chronic and degenerative diseases than ever and that his young patients were coming in with deformed arches, cavities, and crooked teeth. He also noticed a correlation between the number of cavities in a person and disease in their body. Dr. Price was noted for his studies on vibrantly healthy indigenous cultures and their relationship to raw foods. On his travels around the world in the 30's and 40's, he found primitive cultures with superior health and no degenerative diseases such as cancer or heart disease. The diets of these people consisted of raw (sometimes fermented) animal products including raw meats, raw eggs, and raw dairy. The bulk of the raw animal products these cultures consumed included organ meats and meat fat. Organ meats have the highest level of nutrients and some cultures actually discard the muscle meats and consume just the organs.

A physician by the name of Dr. Frances Pottenger was well known for his studies using raw milk with cats. In one of his studies, he fed half of his sick cats raw milk and raw meats, while the other half of his cats were fed the exact same foods, only the meats were cooked and the milk was pasteurized. The cats that were fed the cooked foods developed our modern-day degenerative diseases, while the cats that were fed the raw foods were free of disease generation after generation. Upon autopsy of the cats, the ones on the raw diet had healthy pink organs and strong healthy bones. The cats that ate cooked foods had severe degeneration and deteriorated organs as well as osteoporosis of their bones.

A study by a group of Austrian scientists reported the findings of 812 children as they relate to allergies, asthma and skin problems. 319 of the children had grown up with regular exposure to a farm, including drinking of raw unpasteurized "farm milk". The other 493 were non-farm children. The study found that only 1 % of the farm children showed any signs of asthma as compared to 11% of the non-farm children. 3% of the farm children showed signs of hay fever as compared to 13% of the non-farm children. Children exposed to clean pesticide free soil are healthier than children who do not have this connection to the earth.

Anthropologist, Vilhjalmur Stefansson while living with and studying the Eskimos, noticed they lived on a diet of about 90% raw meat and fish with virtually zero carbohydrates, and were free of our modern-day diseases. He was so convinced that nutritionists were mistaken to recommend the "balanced diet" that we currently know, that he and a fellow explorer, Karsten Anderson, agreed to a study where they ate only meat and water for one year (two pounds of lean meat to a half pound of fat). After one year, Stefansson who had been eating the way Eskimos ate for years remained in excellent health, while Anderson was in far better physical condition and health than when he started the diet.

Side note on elimination:
If anyone has ever transitioned a dog from kibble or cooked food to a 100% raw food diet, one of the first things you will notice is that the size of their poop is significantly reduced. In fact, I had my two 160-pound

Newfoundland's on a raw diet and it was shocking how little waste came out of them. It looked like what you would expect from a small to medium sized dog. The same happens in people. This is because when you cook food you kill it, turning it into waste and that large amount of waste has to be eliminated. When you eat raw food, no matter what the food is, nearly every bit of that food is utilized in the body so there is little waste to be removed.

VITAMINS & SUPPLEMENTS

I am frequently asked about nutritional supplements and if we need them or not. This is an interesting subject because most people do not get the nutrients they need and could use some supplementation. However, most of the supplements on the market today are either synthetic or fractionated, which can cause additional health problems if taken for extended periods of time. Food in its natural state has a complex compound of nutrients including vitamins, enzymes, and trace minerals that all work synergistically together in the body. A specific vitamin is also made up of numerous components and it only works the way it is designed to work when it is complete. When a vitamin company tries to reproduce that vitamin in the lab, it is virtually impossible because of the complex compounds within that are still unknown. A man made, synthetic vitamin, is missing components and is not the way nature created it.

Vitamin supplements sold in stores come in various forms and it is important to understand their differences. There are three basic kinds of vitamins...fractionated, synthetic and whole food vitamins. When a vitamin is sold in its fractionated form, it is not the complex group of compounds found in its whole food form. For example: Vitamin C has over 150 different compounds and yet is not uncommon to find one single component like ascorbic acid or citric acid that has been isolated and sold as "vitamin C". This is not vitamin C. It is one single piece of it. Another example is with vitamin E which is again made of a complex compound of many components, yet alpha tocopherol is commonly sold as vitamin E.

The second kind of vitamin is synthetic, meaning it is man-made in a chemistry lab. Synthetic vitamins are not only man-made, but also fractionated. The only vitamin that is complete is a whole-food vitamin. Not vitamins made by "wholefoods market", a "whole food" vitamin. People really do get that confused. Whole-food vitamins are made from a whole piece of food. For example, cherries, which are high in vitamin C are dried and ground into powder and put into capsules or made into a spray. This is the whole form of vitamin C in the capsule which contains all of its components. Of course it's best to eat the food, but there are times when this is not an option or you need a little boost of a supplement as you may not be getting everything you need. How much vitamins are you really going to get in one little spray or capsule? It may not seem like much, but a little today, and a little the next day, and a little the next day, and a little the next day, accumulates in your body just the same as a toxin would like getting a little lead in your water today, and a little lead in your water the next day, and a little lead in your water the next day...

ENZYMES: A VITAL COMPONENT TO HEALTH

Most people know very little about enzymes other than the fact that they are in our food, but it has been proven that a lack of proper enzymes can lead to some very serious illnesses.

There are three different categories of enzymes: metabolic, digestive and food enzymes. Every organ and tissue in the body depends on metabolic enzymes for survival because they are responsible for repairing damage, and each one has its own specific set of metabolic enzymes designed for its repair. Without these vital metabolic enzymes, organs and tissues could not survive, and eventually the body would not survive.

Digestive enzymes do exactly what the name refers to...they digest the food we eat so the vital nutrients can be assimilated in the body. Where metabolic and digestive enzymes are made within our body, the third category, food enzymes, come from the foods we eat. Food enzymes start food digestion so the body doesn't need to produce so many digestive enzymes to digest the food. Food enzymes are highly susceptible to heat and can be damaged at temperatures as low as 96°F. All cooked and processed foods are completely void of food enzymes. They are destroyed to prevent color changes and preserve the food that would naturally be broken down by the enzymes. This is a huge problem because we each have a fixed amount of enzymes that can be produced by the body in our lifetime called our "enzyme potential". On a raw food diet, the *food enzymes* begin digestion of the food we eat; therefore, few digestive enzymes are needed, leaving ample enzymes in this enzyme pool to be used as metabolic enzymes for running the body.

When we eat cooked food the food enzymes are destroyed causing our body to have to secrete large amounts of digestive enzymes from the pancreas and other digestive organs, causing stress to them and pulling from your total enzyme pool. Now if your organs need metabolic enzymes for repair work to be done, your enzyme pool is depleting itself quickly. If our organs are not being healed and repaired, numerous health problems could occur. On a cooked diet, it is not uncommon to see a weakened and/or enlarged pancreas due to it being overworked. This is one of the main contributing factors to diabetes.

You can see how day after day, and year after year, vital enzymes are being wasted due to all of the cooked and processed foods we ingest. When we are young, we have a large pool of "enzyme potential" to draw from, but as we age and our pool is depleted, eating cooked foods becomes more stressful on the body. A lack of metabolic enzymes in a particular organ or tissue can lead to weakness, disease and even death. Everyone on a standard American diet has disease in the body. It is not always noticeable until later in life but it is there, although it seems debilitating diseases are being diagnosed at younger and younger ages.

Raw nuts, seeds and grains, including raw wheat germ, and raw soybeans contain enzyme inhibitors. When these foods are eaten, the inhibitors cause a great outpouring or wasting of digestive enzymes, again leaving fewer metabolic enzymes to do their healing work. Dr. Edward Howell, a leader in enzyme education and author of "*Enzyme Nutrition*" conducted an experiment where "young rats and chickens were fed a diet of raw soybeans (high in enzyme inhibitors) and huge quantities of pancreatic digestive enzymes were wasted in combating the inhibitors. The pancreas gland enlarged to handle the extra burden, and the animals sickened and failed to grow".

Even when eating cooked food, you can add foods high in digestive enzymes such as raw honey, fresh raw pineapple, mango, banana, avocado or raw kefir to supplement your meal and prevent your body from having to produce them itself.

WATER

Have you ever wondered why all of a sudden, we have to drink so much water? When I was growing up we drank water when we were thirsty and never had to carry around large containers needing to count how many ounces we consumed. What has changed?

One reason is that we are far more toxic than ever before and our body is craving water to try to save our lives. When a toxin or something foreign enters the body, or when the body has an abundance of dead cells, it sends fluids to that area to inflame the area with the purpose of trying to flush it out and heal any damage that happened from the toxin. If you have ever run your hand over some wood and gotten a splinter in it, you noticed that that area swells up around the splinter. The body sends fluids to the area to swell the area so the splinter can be flushed out....or "work is way out". There are blood cells included in this fluid that transport nutrients and oxygen to the area to heal the area that has been traumatized by the toxin or foreign body. All of this requires water. The more toxic the body, the more water is necessary.

Everyone is trying to reduce inflammation in the body, but inflammation has a purpose...to swell up an area to flush out poisons. Stopping inflammation stops the detoxification. If you want to reduce inflammation in your body, reduce the toxins in your system and the inflammation with reduce.

Clean fresh water is a depleting commodity with the growth of our population and the poisoning of our fresh waters. The healthier we get, the less water we need. I do not drink a large amount of water as I get my water through my food, in smoothies, and in juices. When I do drink water, I try to add raw apple vinegar, fresh lemon juice, raw honey, or minerals with Terramin clay so I am at least putting nutrients into the body and not just flushing the out.

On a raw diet your water need is less than someone eating cooked foods. This is because the cooking and dehydrating of food removes the water content. When that person eats the cooked foods, water is pulled from their body to re-hydrate the foods for digestion, thus leeching water from the body. The exception to this is when cooking in water such as when making soups and stews. All raw foods, such as raw eggs, raw meats, raw dairy, fresh raw juices, raw fruits and vegetables, contain water and absolutely count in your daily water intake. Eggs are 80% water and fresh raw muscle meat is up to 75% water. Part of the reason we have to drink so much water today is because we have been falsely told to cook the life out of our food and with it, the water content.

In addition, drinking any kind of liquid with a solid food meal dilutes stomach acids that are necessary to breakdown our foods. If you decrease this breakdown, it disrupts digestion and prevents absorption of the foods and nutrients into the body. How can the nutrients be absorbed if they are not broken down? Taking it a step further, natural bacteria on raw food assists in the breaking down of food and nutrients even further allowing more nutrients to be absorbed.

Yet another reason to eat your food as uncooked as possible.

Naturally sparkling mineral water is a good, relatively clean, source of water to drink as it has, as the bottle says, minerals that help support health. "Naturally sparkling mineral water" comes from the ground with natural carbonation in it and "sparkling natural mineral water" is mineral water with added CO_2 to make it bubbly. Naturally sparkling mineral water with raw honey mixed in is a good remedy for a toxic blood headache. Carbonation increases absorption of the natural minerals.

Bottled spring water comes from a natural spring and contains all of its natural minerals. Nothing has been removed or added. Check the source by calling the company or by checking online as some spring waters are from protected pristine springs and others are from local springs that may have come in contact with agricultural pollutants.

Tap water can come from either a public water system or a well. If it is from a public water system, it has been treated with large amounts of chemicals such as fluoride, chlorine and chloramines, and when chlorine in public water mixes with natural organic matter that is in all public water, the chemical reaction produces a carcinogen called chloroform. Flint, Michigan is not the only city with poisoned public water. All public water has poisons in it which cause harm to the body to some degree. Flint just happened to have a higher level and the impact was seen faster. Everyone drinking public water is also being poisoned and impacted, just more slowly. Disease and chronic illness stem from an accumulation of poisons in the body that harm healthy cells destroying areas and those areas stop functioning the way they are supposed to function.

Well water comes from an aquifer deep below the ground that has been tapped. This water also contains the natural minerals from the earth which are very beneficial to health but should always be tested for chemicals before consumption. Sometimes agricultural or industrial chemicals seep into the ground and over time make their way into the aquifer. It can sometimes have a strong sulfur smell and can be difficult to tolerate by some because of this, but water filtration can remedy some of this problem.

Installing a water purification system is an option for public water systems and is an good choice for public water with the amount of chemicals used to treat it but make sure to be fully educated on the purification system you purchase as some, like reverse osmosis systems, also remove the mineral content and you need to make sure to re-mineralize the water with products such as Terramin clay.

The skin is the largest organ and can absorb large amounts of contaminants. Once they make their way through the skin, most of these toxins make their way directly into the bloodstream where they circulate around the entire body about once every minute. When you take a shower or bath, the chemicals in the water are heated and can turn into a vapor and be even more toxic than the liquid form of the chemical.

Following are just some of the chemicals found in tap water:

- Chlorine
- Chloramine
- Fluoride
- Nitrates
- Pesticides
- Herbicides
- Industrial solvents

Pipes can leech:

- Cadmium
- Lead
- Asbestos

Polyvinyl Chloride (PVC) pipes can leech:

- Methyl Ethyl Ketone (MEK)
- Dimethyl-form amide (DMF)
- Cyclohexanone (CH)
- Tetrahydrofuran (THF)
- Carbon tetrachloride
- Tetrachloroethene
- Trichloroethane
- Dibutyl phthalate
- Vinyl Chloride

These are known carcinogens that cause birth defects, cancer, heart disease, neurological problems, headaches and probably a whole list of issues we don't even know about yet. There is a commercial that used to run when I was a kid showing a pregnant mother standing at the sink in her kitchen drinking a glass of tap water. The voice over says, "a little lead won't hurt me." Then they showed her drinking it over and over and over and over... It is not the one swallow that will hurt anyone; it is the accumulation of toxins from various sources throughout the years over and over that is killing us. That is why it is so important to detoxify and rebuild in some way with some consistency.

Distilled water is another form of purified water but long term use of distilled water can be very dangerous as it has been stripped completely of everything in it, is highly acidic, and will cause every part of your body to leech nutrients, especially electrolytes such as sodium, potassium and chloride as well as trace minerals like magnesium. Does that mean we should never drink it? Of course not. Because it pulls nutrients, it happens to be excellent at pulling the medicinal properties and nutrients from medicinal teas allowing you to drink the tea with the healing herbs in it.

PICK YOUR POISONS

We are exposed to environmental poisons nearly 24/7/365 and there is no longer any place in the world that you can go where you will not be impacted by them to some degree. Understanding the different categories of environmental poisons and becoming aware of what damage they are doing to your physical body is essential so you can increase your awareness and *pick your poisons.*

The goal is to decrease your exposure to environmental poisons so less damage happens to your body and your survival rate as well as the survival rate of your offspring increases, along with your quality of life. Beginning with chemical exposure, decide what you will not give up and what you are willing to give up for your health. The list of options is long.... Shampoos, conditioners, skin care products, deodorants, nail products, shaving creams, lotions, household cleaners, home remodeling products, lawn care products, clothing, auto/boat/rv cleaning products, pesticides/herbicides, insect repellants, air fresheners, food, drinks, water, cookware, storage containers, clothing, furniture, etc... The list goes on.

Below is a short list of chemicals that most of us are exposed to at some level almost daily. All of them are carcinogens, endocrine disruptors, thyroid disruptors, neurotoxins, known to cause birth-defects, kidney and liver disease, reduce IQ, and/or cause behavioral disorders. That is just the damage that we know happens. As I described earlier, once toxins enter the bloodstream, they make a trip around the body once every minute destroying healthy cells along the way until they are excreted from the body, or store in fat or cells or lodged somewhere.

- BPA – Bottles and linings of food cans
- Perfluorinated Compounds (PFC's)- Used on non-stick pans. If your non-stick pan is scratched or you cook at too high of temperatures, the PFC's are being released into your food. Switch to glass cookware. PFC's are also found in paints and stains, firefighting foams, household cleaners, adhesives, and insecticides.
- Atrazine – Pesticide commonly found in drinking water from run-off.
- Organophosphates – Pesticide commonly found in baby food.
- Glycol Ethers – (diethylene glycol dimethyl ether, ethylene glycol monobutyl ether and diethylene glycol monomethyl ether) – Found in cleaning products, liquid soaps, and cosmetics.
- Phthalates – Found in Plastics, Cosmetics and Lotions, toothbrushes, children's toys, insect repellant, water from PVC tubing.
- Perchlorate – Used in Rocket Fuel, Found in our Water
- Arsenic – Found in Water and Rice
- 1,4-Dioxane – Dyes, deodorants, supplements, cosmetics

- Fire Retardants – Found in Mattresses, Upholstered Furniture, and children's pajamas.
- Polyfluoroalkyl substances—or PFAS – Lining of microwave popcorn bags
- Triclosan- Toxic antimicrobial banned from soaps but still being used in toothpaste
- Formaldehyde- (aka: quaternium-15) - Air fresheners, cleaning products, soaps, shampoos, lotions and vaccinations, cabinets, furniture.
- EDTA – Used in food, drinks and cosmetics as a preservative
- Parabens – (aka: benzylparaben, isobutylparaben, butylparaben, ethylparaben and n-propylparaben, benzoic acid, 4-hydroxy-, 2-methylpropyl ester, aseptoform butyl) Skin care, shampoos, deodorants

Get Smart! It goes back to reading labels and empowering yourself with knowledge. Search the internet using key words such as ... "toxicity of xyz". The chemical industry knows that we are educating ourselves and becoming familiar with the names of common poisons so alternative names are given for some. Formaldehyde can be labeled as quaternium-15, and parabens do not necessarily end with the word paraben any longer and can be listed as benzoic acid, 4- hydroxy-, 2-methylpropyl ester, or aseptoform butyl.

TURN DOWN THE HEAT

Change is not easy and we all have powerful food addictions that we face each day. I truly believe that food is the number one addiction in this country. Try eliminating your morning cappuccino or sugar and see what other food replaces that addiction. When you have been eating certain foods for 20, 30, 40 or 50+ years, change takes time. Unlike cigarettes or alcohol, we cannot just stop eating. Similarly, most of us cannot just switch over to a 100% raw diet unless faced with a devastating diagnosis such as cancer and even then, I am astounded at how many people who are given a death sentence or who are in so much physical discomfort will not even try this.

Everyone is different. If you are an extremist like me, you just go for it. I figured, if this is going to make me healthy, I am not going to dilly dally as I want to be as healthy as I can for as long as I can so let's just do it and see what happens. It has personally changed my life and I never turned back. The first couple years I was almost 100% raw to really clean out my body, but now I enjoy my share of cooked foods as well, but almost always with raw fat of some kind such as slathering my toast with raw butter and avocado, or putting heaps of raw butter on my potatoes, or drinking raw unpasteurized dairy with some cooked food that I eat, and I am rarely under 50% raw each day. I would say I average eating 70 – 90% raw most days now. In theory, if you eat 49% cooked and 51%

raw, you are detoxing more than you are putting toxins into the body, but because of the other environmental poisons we are exposed to throughout the day every day, shooting for 70% raw unheated foods a day is exceptional. Anything above 51% is good and moving in the right direction because you counter the 49% cooked food toxins.

It may not be as hard as you think. Start by putting raw unpasteurized milk on your cereal or oatmeal. Doing this gives you nearly a 50/50 ration of raw to processed/cooked. If you truly have the vegetarian gene and you use nut milks, stop buying the processed, heated nut milks (that also frequently have sugar added) from the grocery store and make fresh raw nut milks, or buy them at your local farmer's market.

If you are like the nearly 82% of Americans that *do not* have the vegetarian gene and must eat animal protein for survival, you can grill your hamburger rare so it is not cooked more than 30-40%, add lettuce, which I use in place of a bun as a lettuce wrap, some fresh tomato slices, and fresh onion, and now you are over 50% raw!

Sample meals that are over 50% raw:

Sample Meal 1
- Grilled steak – Seared so only 20 - 30% of steak is cooked. **70-80% raw**
- Salad- **100% raw**
- Salad dressing- Raw unheated olive oil, raw apple cider vinegar, avocado, raw honey, citrus – **100% raw**
- ½ baked sweet potato – **0% raw**

- 2 tablespoons raw unpasteurized butter for potato – **100% raw**

Sample Meal 2 – Ahi Tuna Salad
- Mixed Greens – **100 % raw**
- Seared Fresh Tuna – **80 – 90% raw**
- Avocado for salad – **100% raw**
- Freshly made aioli sauce – **100% raw**
- Homemade dressing – **100% raw**

Sample Meal 3 – Sushi
- Tuna/Avocado/massago rolls – **50 - 80% raw**
- Seaweed salad – **80 – 100% raw**

Sample Meal 4 – Avocado Toast
- Homemade or low ingredient bread/toast – **0% raw**
- Raw butter for toast – **100% raw**
- Avocado – **100% raw**
- Optional lightly poached eggs – **50 – 80% raw**
- Raw sesame seeds – **100% raw**

Sample Meal 5 – Soup
- Homemade broth – **0% raw**
- Sliced raw meat – **50 - 80% raw**
- Warm up some homemade soup broth and drop in slices of raw meat. The broth can be warmed but not so hot that it over cooks the meat.

One of my favorite meals is at Cherry Creek grill in Denver, Colorado. They have an incredible seared tuna salad with avocado. It gives you raw meat (tuna), raw fat (avocado) and raw vegetables all in one meal....detoxing! Lemonade in Los Angeles makes a wonderful tuna poke dish that you can order as a full poke bowl, or as a side dish. When I go to Italian restaurants, I order carpaccio. This is thinly sliced raw beef with olive oil, onions, tomatoes and a little shaved parmesan cheese, which if it is a quality parmesan, is usually made with raw unpasteurized milk. My favorite ceviche' is at a tiny Mexican restaurant in Basalt, Colorado called Taqueria El Nopal and is made with fresh shrimp marinated in lime. This is 100% raw. Detoxing!

INTEGRATION

If we want to move the poisons and debris out of our body and rebuild new healthy cells for health, integrating the following food groups is essential: raw fat, raw protein, fresh vegetable juices, fruits, and nuts and seeds.

1. Raw Fat
   You want a good source of healthy raw fat to be circulating in the blood and body to provide fuel and to absorb toxins that you are consistently exposed to on a daily basis. In addition, they can bond with the toxic fat in the body pulling it out and eventually replacing it with healthy fat.
   Sources include:
      - Raw unpasteurized dairy (raw milk, raw butter, raw cream, rea kefir)
      - Raw eggs
      - Raw fresh coconut cream
      - Avocado
      - Raw unheated nuts and seeds
      - Raw unhated nut and seed oils

2. Raw Protein
   Raw animal protein contains all of the essential amino acids necessary for rebuilding new healthy cells. The body must have all of the necessary amino acids in their complete and natural form to combine together to rebuild

and repair every part of the body. Animal protein includes any type of animal including beef, bison, deer, chicken, turkey and other fowl, all fish and seafood, and all wild game. Vegetarians can also get complete proteins mostly through food combining, but must also be aware of the destruction of amino acids and the production of acrylamides via heat sources. This is important because most vegetarians cook the grain and legume proteins. Doing so produces these toxins I described.

If you are absolutely not available to consume raw animal foods and you do not have the vegetarian gene, you can take raw organ and glandular supplements. These are organs and glands taken from healthy free-range 100% grass-fed animals that are then freeze-dried and put into capsules. Again, there is a gradient to food. Fresh organic grass-fed animal would be best, followed by frozen organic grass-fed, followed by freeze-dried organic grass-fed. You have options.

3. Fruits and Vegetables
    Drinking fresh pressed vegetable juices are the quickest way of getting nutrients to cells in the body as the G.I. tract does not have to break down the cellulose before the nutrients can assimilate into the body. Nutrients from the juice can go directly into the cells. Of course, salads and whole vegetables are absolutely good to eat if you enjoy them.

4. Nuts/Seeds

Raw nuts and seeds can be another excellent food if sprouted and re-dehydrated for crunchy texture, also if not pasteurized or fumigated. Caution: many bodies get stomach cramps and have digestive issues with large amounts of nuts and seeds. If you think about how they come to us in nature, it takes quite a bit of effort to get one small nut out of a shell. It is not logical that we were designed to eat whole meals created from nuts and seeds. That is why so many have difficulty with vegan diets that are based on nuts and seeds. That said, there are those who have the vegetarian allele and whose body has created the enzyme mutations for them. Once again, you must be in touch with your own body and what works best for you. I mention this here because I have had many people tell me that they tried a vegan diet based on nuts and seeds and have had to discontinue because their body did not do well on it. Trust what your body is telling you.

13 EASY WAYS TO INTEGRATE RAW FOODS INTO YOUR CURRENT DIET

1. Replace your current dairy with raw unpasteurized dairy. This includes milk, butter, cream, kefir and yogurt.
2. Morning milkshake – Everyone should drink one of these every day!
3. Smoothies and Orange Julius
4. Eat sushi, carpaccio, ceviche, seared tuna, tuna tartare, steak tartare whenever possible
5. Homemade raw dairy ice cream
6. Homemade popsicles made with raw yogurt and/or avocado as a base.
7. Replace sugar with raw unheated honey
8. Fresh coconut cream – eat with fruit, in smoothies, in ice cream, and in sauces
9. Green Vegetable Juices – fresh pressed juice with a vegetable base
10. Salads – yes a salad counts as raw food. Take note of the toppings you put on it. Are they raw or are your choosing cooked bacon? What about your dressing? Maybe make your own dressing so you know it is raw.
11. Lemon/Cider Honey tea – hot or cold
12. Add Terramin Clay to the liquids you drink
13. Don't change anything in your current diet and pick one thing you can add to what you are doing now such as a green juice, or a morning milkshake. Just make that one

change. Then when you are ready, add a second food that you can do.

Any raw unheated food is better than no raw unheated food. Do what you can and ask your local cafes and restaurants to provide some options for you and again start slow but eventually shooting for a 49/51% cooked to raw ratio **or more**.

As science has taught us about how heat impacts food, and how the higher the temperatures and the longer the food is cooked, the more toxins are created, we can begin by turning down the temperature and decreasing the length of cooking.

Think pure. One way to reduce toxins in food is to start with the purest form of the food. If you bake or cook with butter, make it raw unpasteurized butter. If you start with pasteurized butter, you are starting with butter that has already been heated once and some degree of toxins were created from that first heating process already. Heating it a second time increases the toxicity levels. On the other hand, if you start with raw unpasteurized butter, your cooking will be its first contact with heat...virgin butter! For example, if I were to make cookies with pasteurized butter, the butter will have been heated to high temperatures twice, once during the pasteurization process and once during the baking of the cookies. However, if I make cookies with raw unpasteurized butter, the butter will have only been heated once during the cookie baking. This same principle can be applied to the cooking of any food. Any food that comes in a can has been already heated to preserve the food inside. When cooking, using only ingredients that are in their purest raw form should be the standard practice whenever possible.

The more the food is heated, the more it is processed, the more toxic it is to the body.

People jump on these diets such as vegan, keto, Adkins, or paleo and that is great, but a processed vegan, paleo, or keto snack bar that is made of cooked vegetable oils and highly processed ingredients is still going to damage healthy cells in your body, store toxins in your body, and cause inflammation. French fries are vegan but can cause not only extreme inflammation due to plaque toxins that are created from heating the oil at high temperatures, but also acrylamides from cooking the potato starch at high temps.

The closer food is to its true nature the healthier it is.

TERRAMIN CLAY

Terramin clay is a calcium montmorillonite living clay that functions in three ways: it adds macro, micro and trace minerals to the body, it has a negative ionic charge that binds with the positive ionic charge of toxins, and it alkalizes the blood neutralizing the toxins.

Unlike many other types of clay, it has a particle size that is small enough to allow it to pass through the blood barrier and cell membrane to get the nutrients inside of your cells. It is one thing to ingest clay that has a high amount of nutrients in it, but Terramin clay can also get those nutrients inside the cells to nourish and cleanse them. We know that vitamins will not function properly without trace elements and that enzymes are activated by trace elements, so it is crucial to get them in our diets. Because modern day farming has significantly depleted much of the trace elements from our soil, it is important to supplement them in our diets. Modern day diets that are so void of minerals we really do need the added support of Terramin clay.

Terramin clay also has a negative ionic charge that supports the removal of toxins in the body by bonding with the positively charged poisons, allowing them to be eliminated efficiently. If you look at the clay under a microscope it looks kind of like a sponge with a porous structure. If you were to wipe a sponge over a counter with spilled grape juice, the grape juice would get sucked up into the sponge through the pores. This is the same kind of action that occurs with Terramin clay. Toxins get absorbed into the clay through the pores and are held there as it passes through the body. Studies at Cal Tech University show that Terramin clay has the three perfect components that allow it to be easily absorbed into the cells. It has a particle size of 10-20 microns (smallest available), it has an open negative ionic state, and it has the perfect ratio of minerals.

Terramin clay has no taste but is a bit gritty. After all, it is 13-million year-old dirt. It comes in powder form which can be put in your juices, smoothies, water or sauces. It is especially good to use in juices that are made of vegetables and fruits that are not organic to absorb the pesticides that were sprayed on the produce. I have even put a little clay in popsicles, ice cream, and chocolate puddings that I have made to give the food a little extra detoxification effect.

Note: For full disclosure, the tablets and caplets are pressed together with a tiny amount of oil that is not raw.

CLOSING WORDS

I am often asked questions like, "What if I really want a cup of coffee?" My response is, "Have a cup of coffee." My goal here is to provide you with knowledge and to heighten your awareness. I am not asking you to completely change your life, unless you are very ill and then you may have to make more extreme changes to save your life. If you have tried everything the medical community has to offer or have been given a death sentence, the medical community cannot do anything else for you. Why would you not try this? I know many people who were given death sentences and are alive today because they switched to a raw diet that included raw fat and raw animal protein to detoxify their body and rebuilt healthy new cells.

We were designed to live in nature with nature and to eat natural foods in their purest form. The food pendulum has swing so far away from what is real food with all of the processed and preserved foods on the shelves, that our views have become distorted as to what is "normal". Just look at the typical grocery store. There was a time when a grocery store meant meat, dairy, produce, and some basic staples. Now, we have aisles and aisles and aisles of overly processed foods with a list of ingredients a mile long.

I went into my local grocery store the other day to buy a loaf of bread. There was the traditional bread aisle, and there was a bread section with what looked like artisan loaves of bread, and there was a section of bread under the deli counter, and there was a specialty bread section at the end of an aisle. I spent about 15 minutes reading ingredients looking for just one loaf that said wheat, water, salt. No matter what section I went to, loaf after loaf after loaf had chemicals and preservatives. All I wanted was a loaf of bread made from the 5 basics. But it was not to be found. Instead, every one of them had ingredients including some of the following:

- Ammonium Sulfate- used to regulate acidity. Made by treating ammonia, often a by-product from coke ovens, with sulfuric acid.
- Azodicarbonamide (ADA)- this chemical creates semicarbazide (SEM) during bread making which has been shown to increase the incidence of tumors.
- Potassium Bromate- known to cause kidney and thyroid tumors.
- Butylated Hydroxyanisole (BHA) – known to cause cancer.
- Carmel Coloring – produces 2- and 4-methylimidazole (2- or 4-MEI) during processing and are known to cause cancer.
- High Fructose Corn Syrup – Researches at the Univesity of Utah found it to be more toxic than sugar.
- Soy (Soy oil or soy lecithin) – Approximately 80% of soy on the market is genetically modified.

- Calcium Propionate (preservative) – proven to induce inflammation, stomach ulcers and cause behavioral disturbances in children.
- Thiamine Mononitrate- a synthetic (chemical form) of vitamin B1.
- Sodium Stearoyl – used as an emulsifier. Not much known about toxicity except risk of uterine polyps if taken consistently.
- Hydrogenated & Partially Hydrogenated Oils – Linked to heart disease, diabetes, and stroke.
- Natural & Artificial Flavors: Monosodium glutamate can be listed on food labels as "natural flavors", while artificial flavorings have long been known to damage healthy cells in the body.

I finally found one brand made by Stone House Bread that is made of 4 simple ingredients: organic unbleached wheat flour, well water, sea salt, and malted barley flour. We have gotten so far away from real food in its true nature, that we look at people like myself eating what we were designed to eat, and I am the one called "crazy". Our discernment of what is healthy and unhealthy has completely fallen off track with the bulk of grocery store foods being processed.

You will be amazed at how good you feel when you start transitioning raw and minimally cooked foods into your diet. Even if you eat one raw meal a day, at least you are getting a high dose of nutrition and detoxing your body instead of putting poisons into your body for that one meal. Some is better than none. I present this information so that you can understand how our toxic environment is impacting us heavily and causing these severe health issues. It is not bacteria and viruses that are the problem, it is the host that is the problem. Clean up the host and you clear up disease.

Sometimes hearing information like what I have presented is very difficult, because accepting what I say to be true means everything you have been told is a lie and much of what you have been providing for yourself and your family is unhealthy. It is not that it has all been a lie as much as it has been misinformation. Doctors are not intentionally trying to deceive you, they have not been given all of the information themselves. They have done an exceptional job with what they have had to work with. It is like raising children. We do the best we can based on how we were raised and what information our parents gave to us. Then we become parents and gain additional knowledge and new information that makes us better parents. To quote the great late Maya Angelou, "Sometimes we do things because we don't know better, but once we know better, we can do better".

Our food is an energy source and we have the choice to put life or death into our bodies. Our body already has enough of your own dead cells from all the poisons you have come in contact with, it doesn't need you to put more death into it. Death creates death and Life Creates Life! Choose to live!

Eat lots of healthy raw fat, uncooked meat, and fresh pressed vegetable juices to support your health and wellness.

Do your best when you can. I tell clients to work out every day because there is always going to be something that comes up where you will not be able to. The same goes with food. Eat clean, healthy and as much uncooked as you can when you can because there will always be events, parties, holidays, vacations, or just days when you choose not to. This helps keep you in balance. You will notice a difference if you just try. Truly make an effort.

PANACEA

In my book, *Panacea,* I go into greater depth about the different types and categories of environmental poisons in addition to chemical and physical poisons that impact us. The human being is made of 6 basic components ... the physical body, our mind, our spirit, our emotions, our energy, and our connections to ourselves and the Universe. Each of these components has its own level of toxins which cause destruction and actual death of healthy cells in the body. All of these aspects of who we are and how we are connected in the universe are themselves all connected, and traits are passed from generation to generation.

Most of the time we are looking for "the answer" to a disease, but not only are diseases caused by toxins & deficiencies, but these toxins and deficiencies come from the different aspects of who we are as human beings in addition to the toxins and deficiencies from the depths of our connections to those around us in the world. I know it sounds complicated but in my book Panacea and on my website, I show some very clear diagrams that help understand this concept.

The following is an example of how an emergency surgery was created from multiple toxic components of several human beings all intersecting and impacting one young 24 year old woman. I have a client who as a child, did not feel love and warmth from her mother. The mother had brought in toxic emotions and mental thinking from previous experiences of sexual abuse from her own childhood which created a mental barrier in her, and a physical barrier between her and her own daughter. This negatively impacted the daughter who felt rejected by her mother causing her stress from this relationship which negatively impacted her physical body causing discomfort in her body. She noticed that when she was ill, she got attention from her mother so she began creating stories of having stomach aches and not feeling well so she could stay home from school and have time alone with her mother. The mother had fallen heavily onto the pharmaceutical bandwagon which was pushed by her family physician, who, as a side note, happened to be a very handsome man. The mother, attracted to the family doctor had no problem taking her daughter in to see this handsome man every time she made up the stomachache story as she did not have a fulfilling relationship with her husband and she enjoyed the connection with this doctor.

Each time the mother did this, the little girl was given a full round of antibiotics which she took. We know from studies that it takes only 4 days to completely eradicate the trillions of gut bacteria leaving no bacteria and microbes to protect the gut from the medications being taken, thus causing IBD, colitis, Crohn's disease, polyps, and other G.I. disorders including the thinning of the G.I. tract. Over the years, the G.I. tract of this girl became very weak and thinned out. The stomachache story she created in her mind actually created a real stomach problem. The girl grew to be a beautiful young woman who continued the antibiotic use into adulthood. She married a man who ended up being a combination of her mother and father (an alcoholic like her father and jealous like her mother). She divorced after only about a year of marriage. The stress of a newborn, being with an abusive alcoholic man, and a hypercritical mother, added to the G.I. issues she experienced. After the divorce she dated and drank alcohol heavily because of the pressure from a man she dated and girlfriends.

The young woman went in to see her family doctor for stomach aches and he did a colonoscopy on her. The weakened intestinal lining from heavy antibiotics, stress, and alcohol, lead to the physician perforating her colon. She was rushed into the hospital where her rectum, colon and large intestine were removed, and an ileostomy was performed at 24 years old.

Disease and medical issues are complicated. What was the cause of this young woman to have an ileostomy? We want an easy answer but there are no easy answers. We want to point to one thing as a cause, but there is never only one cause. The cause of every disease is an accumulation of environmental toxins and deficiencies. In this case the toxins were: the toxic reactive mind and emotions of a mother that impacted this young girl/woman emotionally causing stress that impacted her body, the over prescribing of antibiotics and other medications by the family physician, the toxic marriage to an abusive alcoholic man, the deficiency of not being able to say "no" to peer pressure to drink, and an unnecessary colonoscopy.

The **only** way to health and wellness is for each of us to be on a consistent detoxification and rebuilding program of all of these aspects of who and what we are as human beings. Each of us impacts the health of every other person we are in contact with. I may live a clean life and choose to not use chemicals in my home, but when I visit a friend's home or stay with another person who uses harsh chemicals in their home, their choices now impact my physical body. Someone who has a reactive mind and blows up on the highway at another driver can cause an accident to other innocent people on the road. We are each responsible for detoxing all of the aspects of our own being ... body, mind, soul, emotions, energy and connections to the world. My book Panacea, goes into this in greater detail.

SUMMARY

Whatever your belief.... The creation of the earth by
God, or the science of evolution, makes no difference.
This is the world that we were designed to live in......
in nature with nature. With all of its biomes.

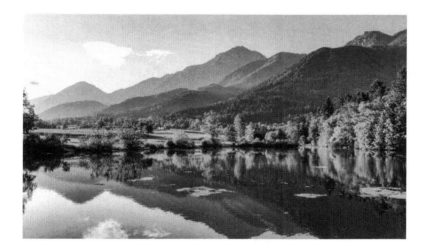

Not the toxic world we have created.

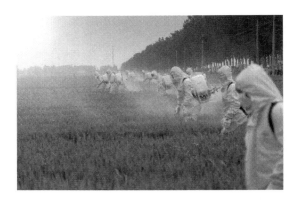

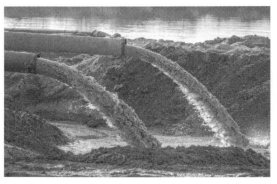

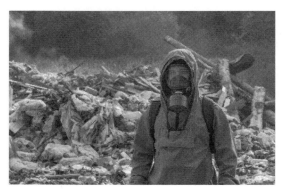

When environmental toxins enter our body, they destroy healthy cells leaving cellular debris and cell corpses along with the toxins.

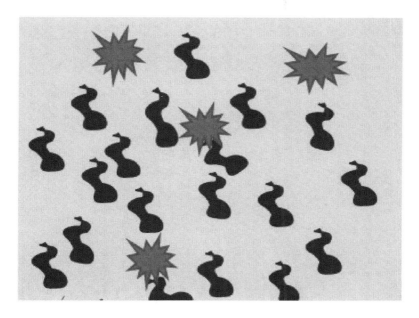

Our bodies were naturally designed to remove toxins and cellular debris and when we have an accumulation of them, our body uses and/or creates a bacteria, virus, parasite or mold to breakdown these toxins, cell corpses, and debris so it can move all of this garbage out of us efficiently. Similar to how bacteria breaks down vegetation in a compost pile.

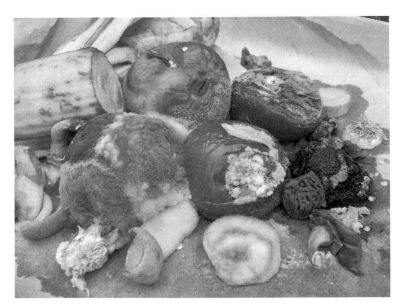

"Symptoms" such as diarrhea, vomiting, fever/sweating, phlegm, coughing, runny nose, watery eyes, skin eruptions, and other bacterial and viral symptoms are actually the body riding itself of these poisons.

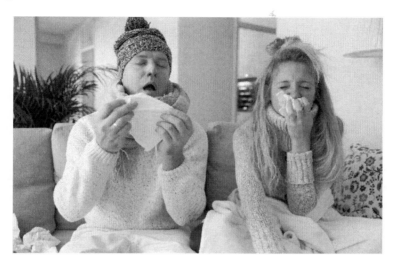

We have scientific studies from major medical institutions to prove it.

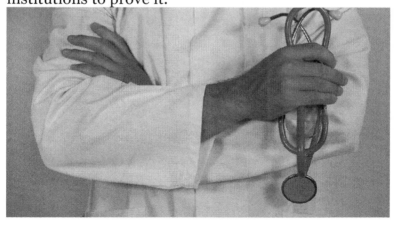

Because of this world we have created, we have too many toxins, cell corpses, and debris in our body causing **Toxic Body Overload**. We are poisoning ourselves to cancer, and to heart disease, and to lupus, and to diabetes, and to asthma, and to dementia, and to birth defects, and to arthritis, and to autism, and to death.

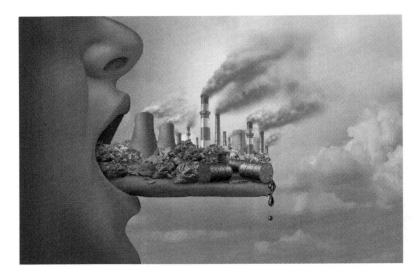

A problem occurs because we have been conditioned to believe that bacteria and viruses are bad and to destroy them as soon as their "symptoms" begin, so we take medications to stop the symptoms and push the toxins back into the body, and add additional toxins from the synthetic medication which can do additional damage to the body.

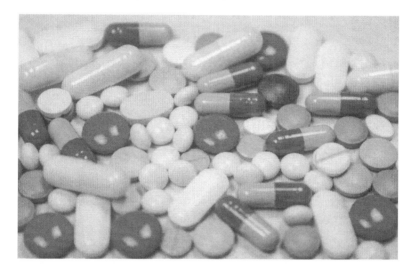

The cause of disease is not microbes but environmental toxicity & deficiencies. It is the toxicity of the HOST that causes disease and determines how intense the detoxification is and how long it lasts.

Some detoxifications are much too intense for some people to go through all at once because their body is so toxic. In cases like this, medications can be used to stop or reduce the detoxification process.

If you choose to stop or prevent the detoxification process with medications, you must understand that you are stopping poisons from exiting the body plus you are adding additional synthetic medications, and in the case of vaccinations you are also adding chemical poisons (see CDC website for a complete list of chemical in vaccinations). So, you must find another way to detoxify these poisons so they do not cause disease in the body. Otherwise, they stay in the body and cause ongoing disease.

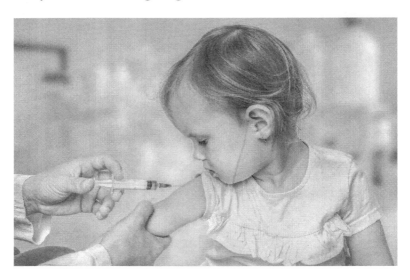

Usually people associate the word "detox" with drug and alcohol detox only, but detoxification means the removal of all matter that is toxic to the physical body. There are several ways to actually physically remove toxins from the body.

The first thing to do is to turn off the faucet. Choose what poisons you are going to allow into your personal body and discard the others. If you live together as a family, decide together what you can get rid of. ie: using clean non-toxic cleaning products in the home, or choosing wood toys instead of plastic toys that go into the mouths of babies, using non-toxic home décor products such as paints and stains, using non-toxic pest control, organic foods, etc

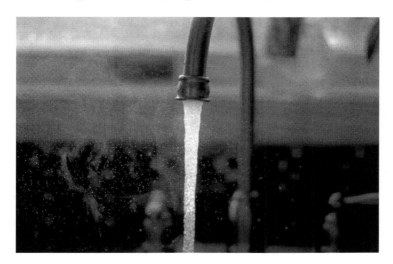

Eat raw foods. All food in its purest unheated raw form has a negative ionic charge to it. Toxins have a positive ionic charge to them. The negative charge from the raw food attracts the positive charge of the toxins as it passes through the body to pull them out. *NOTE: Cooking food creates a toxic positive ionic charge and it no longer detoxes the body. In addition, it deposits toxins such as dead cells, acrylamides, heterocyclic amines, and lipid peroxides. So any food you put in your body that is unheated detoxes your body.

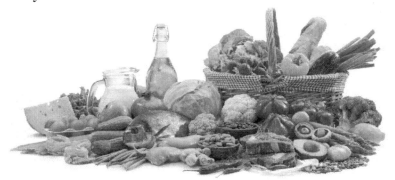

Examples of raw food include: Sushi, Ceviche, Carpaccio, Kibbe, Beef or Tuna Tartare, Raw Unpasteurized Dairy (milk, cream, butter, yogurt, kefir, cheese), eggs, fresh fruits/vegetables and their fresh pressed juices, un-steamed and unheated grains, unpasteurized/unroasted nuts and seeds, unprocessed nut and seed oils (caution with oils as many use chemical or high temperature extraction to make the oil).

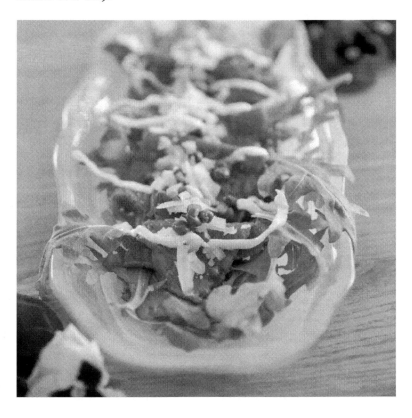

Make healthy raw fat a TOP priority. Getting healthy raw fat into your bloodstream protects your body from the poisons you are exposed to every day. If you are going to have surgery and having medications injected into your body, you want fat to protect your brain and body. If you are going to expose yourself to any form of toxin, you want raw fat in your bloodstream to protect you. If you are going to drink alcohol, eat raw fat first. If you smoke, eat raw fat to help absorb some of the smoking toxins. If you are going to choose to use caustic household cleaning chemicals, eat raw fat. Eat raw FAT, FAT, and FAT.

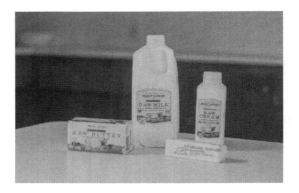

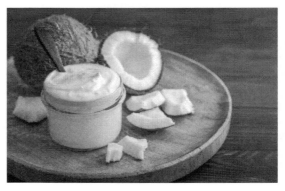

Bacteria: Raw foods also have natural bacteria that predigest your food, and breakdown debris in your body to pass out as the food passes out. Eating raw food that has small amounts of bacteria allow your body to do frequent mini-detoxes so you don't have to go through huge viral and bacterial detoxifications.

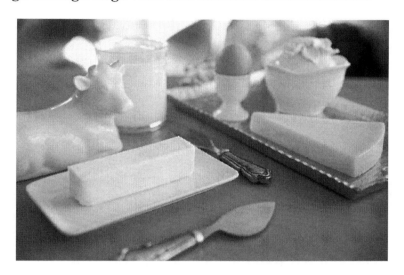

If you cannot or will not eat it completely raw, the less it is cooked the better such as eating a steak seared or rare as opposed to well done, or lightly steaming vegetables as opposed to grilling them. There is a gradient to toxicity in food determined by how long and at what temperature the food has been cooked in addition to what the animals ate or how the food was grown and processed.

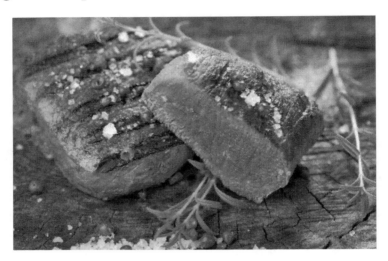

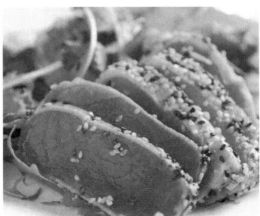

The Law of 51%. If you are eating 51% raw unheated foods and 49% cooked foods, in theory you are eating more raw/uncooked than cooked thus detoxing more than you put into your body.

Terramin Clay is 13 million-year-old clay that also has a negative ionic charge. When ingested, it binds with the positive ionic charge of toxins. It has a porous structure and pulls the toxins into the center like a sponge holding them there until it is passed out of the body. It also has a micron size which is so small it can pass the blood barrier getting inside of cells and circulating through the entire body to cleanse it while also adding valuable micronutrients to the body.

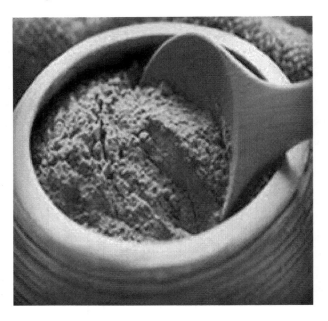

Sweat. Studies show that sweating can remove more heavy metals than the kidneys can through urine. Sweating can flush out the lymphatic system. Find a way to sweat...sports, hot yoga, sauna, steam rooms, hot tubs, hot baths, and sex.

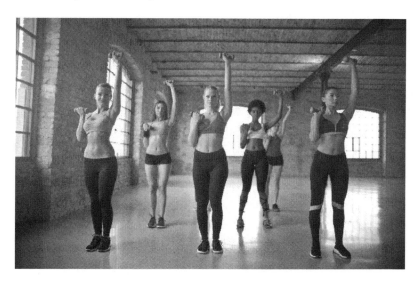

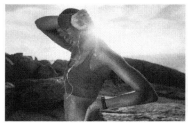 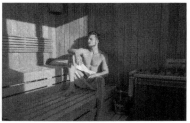

As I mentioned, toxicity is one of the causes of disease. Deficiencies are the other. Raw foods have the highest nutrient level and feed your cells strengthening them. Again, when you cook food, you create toxins you are putting in your body and you are reducing the nutrient level of the food you are putting in your body. If toxicity and deficiencies lead to disease, the opposite is true. Raw unheated foods are non-toxic, provide high levels of nutrients, and detoxify.

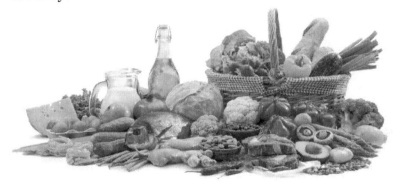

The human being is made of 6 basic components ...
the physical body, our mind, our spirit, our emotions,
our energy, and our connections to ourselves and the
world. Each of these components has its own level of
toxins which cause actual death of healthy cells in the
body. The **only** way to health and wellness is to be on
a consistent detoxification and rebuilding program of
all of these aspects of who and what we are. This is the
only way to get to the root of health and wellness.

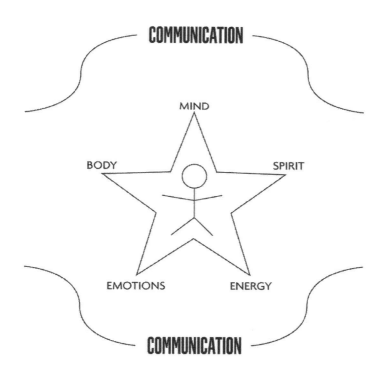

RECIPES

Milk Shakes

- 2-3 Raw Eggs (fertilized if accessible)
- 12 - 14 oz Raw Unpasteurized Milk
- 1 Tbl Raw Unheated Honey

Blend these three ingredients until honey is mixed in, then add desired flavors.
I like to use frozen fruit so it makes the milkshake thicker and nice and cold

Suggested milkshake flavor options:
Cinnamon – Banana: whole frozen banana and teaspoon organic cinnamon
Strawberry – Banana: ½ to 1 frozen banana and frozen strawberries
Banana – Blueberry: ½ to 1 frozen banana and 1 cup frozen blueberries

Raw Milk Coffee/Latte/Cappuccino

If you make your own coffee at home, one of the best things you can do is to switch to raw unpasteurized milk. Roasted coffee has cancer causing acrylamides in it. Making an iced latte with raw milk allows the raw fat in the milk and cream to bond with the toxins in the espresso shot which will protect your body.

Avocado Seaweed Rolls (kids love these)

- Large sheets of raw seaweed
- 1 Avocado
- Sea salt or pink Himalayan salt

Fold seaweed in half creasing the fold. Tear the two pieces apart. Fold each of these in half again and tear apart so the one large piece has now made 4 small pieces. Cut your avocado in half and with a spoon scoop out small pieces and place in the center of the seaweed from one end to the other. Sprinkle avocado with salt. Roll seaweed up like a sushi roll and serve.

Basic Green Juice

- 1 whole stalk of Celery
- 2 Cucumbers
- Spinach
- ½ - 1 Apple
- ½ Lemon (rind cut off)
- Thumb size piece Fresh Ginger
- Optional 4 ounces Raw Milk or 2 Tbl coconut cream

Juice celery, cucumber, spinach, and apple, then pour through a strainer to separate the pulp. Cut off lemon rind and put the lemon and ginger through the juicer. Pour into strained green juice. Store juice in large canning jars.

Option: When you are ready to drink the juice pour about 8 ounces into blender with 4-6 ice cubes. Add 4 ounces raw milk or coconut cream and blend. The raw fat will help bind with toxins being pulled out by the fresh juice and for me the milk softens the taste of the drink making it more palatable.

Lemon - Cider Honey Tea/Drink

- Juice of ½ Lemon
- 1 Tablespoon Raw Apple Cider Vinegar
- 1 Heaping Tablespoon Raw Honey
- Cayenne pepper (optional)

Warm water just enough so you can put your finger in it without burning it. Add your ingredients listed above and enjoy!
*I also put this same mixture in naturally sparkling spring water for a cooler refreshing drink.

Coconut Lemonade

- 8 – 12 oz Fresh Coconut Water from young white coconut
- ½ Small Lime, peeled
- ½ Small Lemon, peeled
- 1 Heaping Tablespoon Raw Unheated Honey

Blend all ingredients in blender until honey mixed in well. Add 1 cup or more of ice and blend again. Enjoy this delicious, refreshing drink!

Note: Using fresh coconut water from a young white Thai coconut will yield the most water and will have the highest nutrient level. There are also some fresh raw coconut waters now available in bottles but all have gone through some degree of pasteurization. Many claim to be raw but use HPP (high pressure pasteurization) where pressure is used instead of heat to destroy bacteria and microbes. The purpose of eating fresh foods is to get the natural bacteria into the body for detoxification purposes if possible. When making fresh coconut cream, you can save the water from inside the brown coconuts to use in smoothies or to make coconut lemonade.

Smoothies/Smoothie Base
- 2-3 Raw Eggs
- ½ Cup Raw Milk
- 1-2 Tbl Raw Yogurt, Raw Coconut Cream or Raw Cow Cream
- 1 Tbl Raw Honey

Blend all base ingredients in a blender then add frozen fruit of choice. Sample Flavors below.

Tropical Smoothie:
- ¼ cup Fresh Squeezed Orange Juice
- ½ Frozen or Fresh Banana
- ½ Cup Frozen Strawberries
- ½ Cup Frozen Mango

Strawberry / Pineapple Smoothie:
- 1 Cup Frozen Strawberries – sliced
- 1 Cup Frozen Pineapple - sliced

Blueberry / Banana Smoothie:
- 1 Frozen Banana
- 1 Cup Frozen Blueberries

Strawberry / Banana Smoothie:
- ½ - 1 Frozen Banana
- 1 Cup Sliced Frozen Strawberries

Mixed Berry Smoothie:
- 1 Cup + Frozen Strawberries, Blueberries, Blackberries, and Raspberries.

Orange Julius

I use this one for the onset of illness

- 2-3 Raw Eggs
- 1 Tbl Raw Unheated Honey
- Juice of 3-4 fresh Organic Oranges
- 2 Tbl Cow Cream or Coconut Cream

Blend all ingredients in blender until honey is mixed in well. Add equal amount of ice and blend in blender until thick and frosty.

At the onset of cold/flu or fever, drink this smoothie, take a hot bath, put some pure lavender oil on your feet and get a good night sleep in a dark room. This elixir seems to speed up the detox and recovery process.

Wild Shrimp & Salmon Ceviche'

- ½ lb fresh wild salmon
- ½ lb wild shrimp
- 2 limes

  Sauce:
- ¼ qt cherry tomatoes sliced in half
- ¼ - 1/3 jalapeno pepper finely diced
- ½ " slice red onion – finely diced
- Thumb size piece fresh ginger – peeled and finely diced
- ½ bunch fresh cilantro – cut off stems and dice leaves into small pieces
- ½ - 1 whole avocado – diced into approx. ¾" chunks
- ¼ cup Unheated olive oil
- ¼ cup Raw apple cider vinegar
- 4-6 limes
- 2-3 tablespoons raw unheated honey

Cut up fish into small 1/2 inch pieces and marinate in lime juice. Let sit in refrigerator while you are making the sauce. Ok to let marinate a few hours or overnight.
Chop jalapeno, red onion, ginger, tomato and cilantro and place into bowl. You can never have too much cilantro!
Pour equal amounts raw apple cider vinegar & olive oil...just enough to cover top of ingredients.
Add raw honey and mix well.
Cut avocado into chunks and mix in last so it does not get mushy. I like large chunks of avocado & tomato.
Pour lime juice off of fish and place fish into serving bowl. Mix sauce into fish.
For smaller appetizer portions, serve in empty avocado halves.
Serves 1-2, 3-5 appetizer portions
Everyone loves this dish. This is a great recipe for those starting a raw diet.

Tenderloin Appetizer

- Fresh Beef Tenderloin
- 1 Medium Tomato
- Raw Unsalted Cheese
- Fresh Basil
- Balsamic Vinegar

Slice tenderloin cross grain into small thin pieces. Slice tomato into thin slices then slice the slice in half so it looks like a half pizza. Layer steak into tomato slice then top with grated or sliced raw cheese and a basil leaf. Arrange several on tray and drizzle balsamic vinegar over all of them. I like to arrange the appetizers on a white tray and drizzle the balsamic in a back and forth pattern for a beautiful presentation.

Beef Carpaccio with Goat Cheese

- Fresh Beef Tenderloin
- Goat Cheese
- Chives chopped into small pieces
- Balsamic Vinegar
- Pink Himalayan Salt

Slice tenderloin cross grain in thin slices. Take a piece of goat cheese about the size of your thumb and shape it like an oval shape. Lay it on one of the tenderloin slices and roll it up. Repeat using all of tenderloin and goat cheese. Sprinkle chives and salt over each rolled beef/cheese roll. Drizzle balsamic over the top.

Buffalo Tartar

- 1 lb - Ground Buffalo
- ¼ quart Cherry Tomatoes – chopped
- ½ - 1 Jalapeno pepper – diced
- Red Onion – equal to jalapeno, diced
- 1 tsp Fresh Ginger – diced
- 4 Fresh Basil Leaves – chopped
- ¼ - 1/3 cup Raw Apple Cider Vinegar
- ¼ - 1/3 cup Virgin or Extra Virgin Olive Oil 1 Tablespoon Raw Unheated Honey
- ½ to 1 Avocado
- Pink Himalayan Salt or Sea Salt

Place ground buffalo in bowl.
Sauce:
Put tomato, jalapeno, red onion, ginger and basil into separate bowl.
Pour in equal amounts olive oil and apple cider vinegar; enough to almost cover vegetables.
Add raw honey and mix well.
Add avocado into sauce last.
Mix sauce into beef and serve.
You can use circular molds to form.
Garnish with fresh tomato and avocado slices and sprinkle with sea salt

Chicken Ceviche'

- 1 Large Whole Chicken Breast

  Sauce:
- ¼ of a Jalapeno Pepper
- ¼ inch slice of a Red Onion
- ¼ quart of Cherry Tomatoes
- 2" square chunk Raw Unsalted Cheese
- 10 Fresh Basil Leaves
- ½ - 1 Whole Avocado

Cut a whole boneless, skinless chicken breast into small pieces , about 1" squares and put in a bowl.
Cover the chicken with enough fresh lemon juice to cover the top. Let marinade while preparing sauce.
In separate bowl make sauce with tomato, jalapeno, red onion, ginger and basil.
Pour in equal amounts olive oil and apple cider vinegar, enough to almost cover vegetables.
Add raw honey and mix well.
Add avocado into sauce last.
Mix sauce into chicken and serve.
Pour 1/8 cup of raw apple cider vinegar over chicken.
Add 1/8 cup virgin olive oil to chicken. Add ingredients you cut up. Mix well. Add 2-3 heaping tablespoons raw unheated honey. Mix well and enjoy.

Avocado Custard

- 1 Raw Egg
- 1 Avocado
- 1 Tablespoon Coconut Cream or Cow Cream
- 1 Tablespoons Raw Unheated Honey (or to taste)
- Optional ½ banana
- Dried coconut flakes
- Ground cinnamon

Put all ingredients in blender and blend until creamy. Top with coconut flakes and cinnamon

Note: Some people have more difficulties digesting avocados than others. If they create a lot of gas, back off on the frequency that you eat them. In my experience, people who do not digest avocados well, do better with animal fats such as raw milk and raw cream. Test it out and see how your body does.

Chocolate Avocado Custard
(option: Freeze in Popsicle Molds)

- 1 Raw Egg
- 1 Avocado
- 1 Tablespoon Coconut Cream or Cow Cream
- 2 Tbl Raw Cacao Powder (for stronger chocolate flavor increase this amount)
- 2 Tbl Raw Unheated Honey
- ½ Fresh Banana (the more ripe it is the sweeter it will taste)
- Ground Cinnamon – for topping
- Coconut Flakes – for topping

Put all ingredients in blender and blend until creamy. The addition of the raw cacao makes the pudding bitter so the more cacao you add, the more raw honey you may need to add. Top with dried coconut flakes and ground cinnamon.

Peach Ice Cream

- 1 Raw Egg
- 1 cup Fresh Raw Cow Cream
- 1 cup Fresh Unpasteurized Milk
- 1 Heaping Tablespoon Raw Unheated Honey
- 2 Peeled Fresh Organic Peaches

Mix ingredients in blender and place in ice cream maker.
If you are using frozen peaches, make sure to mix egg, cream and honey first so honey can blend into mixture well. Then, add frozen fruit.
Serving size: 2-3

Banana Ginger Ice Cream

- 1 Raw Egg
- 1⁄4 - 1/3 qt Fresh Raw Cow Cream
- 1 Heaping Tablespoon Raw Unheated Honey
- 1 Peeled Banana
- 1 tsp Fresh Ginger Juice – juiced in juicer

Mix ingredients in blender and place in ice cream maker. Serving size: 2-3

Banana Cream Pie

- Crust:
  2 – 4 oz Raw Pecans
- 2 – 4 oz Raw Walnuts
- 2 Tbl Shredded Dried Coconut
- 1 Raw Egg
- 1 Tbl Raw Butter – room temperature
- 1 Tbl Raw Unheated Honey

Pulse nuts in blender until they are small chunks then pour into mixing bowl. In separate small mixing bowl, beat egg butter and honey. Put coconut into dry ingredient bowl and mix together with spoon or spatula. Pour wet ingredients into dry and hand mix with spoon. Add more honey to taste if needed.

- Banana Filling:
  Ripe bananas
- Raw Honey
- 1 teaspoon lemon juice
  Mash ripe bananas with a fork until mush. Mix in lemon juice and raw honey to taste.

Topping:
Raw Cream
Raw Honey
Mix a small amount of honey (to taste) with the cream and whip with a hand mixer until firm.
Layer as follows: Crust, filling and topping.
Make small individual servings or one large serving.
Serve immediately or refrigerate for 1/2 to 1 hour before serving.

Chocolate Macaroons

- 4 cups medium shredded dried coconut
- 1 ¼ cups raw cacao powder
- ¼ teaspoon Himalayan salt

- 1 ¼ cups raw unheated honey
- 4 Tablespoons raw unrefined coconut oil
- 1 Tablespoon vanilla

Combine wet and dry ingredients in two separate bowls and mix each bowl of ingredients well. Pour wet ingredients into bowl of dry ingredients and mix well. Using a small teaspoon, scoop a small amount onto cookie sheet. Do not roll macaroon into a tight ball. Just kind of scoop some out and make a small mound. Refrigerate. Keep refrigerated.

Raw Overnight Oats

- 2 ½ Cups Overnight Oats
- ½ Cup Chia Seeds
- 4 Cups Raw Unpasteurized Milk (or Fresh Homemade Coconut Milk)
- ½ Cup each Blueberries, Strawberries, Blackberries, Raspberries
- 2 Tbl Raw Unheated Honey
- Sliced or Chopped Raw Almonds

Put oats and chia seeds into large mixing bowl and mix the two dry ingredients. In blender blend together milk and 1 Tablespoon raw honey on low speed to mix in honey. Add ¼ cup of each of the berries and blend again making a berry milk. Pour milk and berry mixture into mixing bowl and mix all ingredients. Pour or ladle out mixture into bowls or wide mouth jars. Top with remainder of mixed berries and almond slices and refrigerate overnight. In the morning drizzle with raw honey and serve.

Banana Chia Pudding

- 4 large ripe bananas
- 18 ounces raw unpasteurized milk (or fresh coconut milk)
- 1 ½ teaspoons vanilla extract
- ½ teaspoon lemon juice
- ¼ teaspoon Himalayan Salt
- 2 tablespoons raw unheated honey (or to taste)
- 6 1/2 Tablespoons chia seeds
- ¼ cup shredded dried coconut
- Ground cinnamon

In blender mix raw milk, bananas, vanilla, salt and honey on low to medium speed until blended well. Add chia seeds and blend on low speed until seeds are well combined. About 10 seconds. Pour into large bowl and put a layer of parchment paper or plastic wrap on the top of mixture to prevent a film from forming. Chill overnight. In glass jars or glasses, fill about 1/3rd of the jar with chilled mixture. Add a layer of sliced bananas and a sprinkle of coconut. Add another layer of chia pudding, sliced bananas and coconut. Sprinkle top with ground cinnamon.

REFERENCES

Abrams, Jr., H. Leon, (1982),"Anthropological Research Reveals Human Dietary Requirements for Optimal Health", Journal of Applied Nutrition, 16:1:38-45

American Cancer Society, "Acrylamide and Cancer Risk, What is Acrylamide?", www.cancer.org. Bon Appetit Magazine, 15 Raw Meat Dishes From Around The World, www.bonappetit.com

Cohen, D. Paul, Vonderplanitz, Aajonus,"Can we prevent and cure most diseases by nutrition?" Cohen Independent Research Group

Cousins, Gabriel (2000), "Conscious Eating".

Dadd, Debra Lynn (1997) "Home Safe Home", New York, NY: Penguin/Putnam

DeCava, Judith A. (1997) "The Real Truth About Vitamins & Antioxidants"

Deoni SC[1], Zinkstok JR[2], Daly E[2], Ecker C[2]; MRC AIMS Consortium, Williams SC[3], Murphy DG[2]. "White-matter relaxation time and myelin water fraction differences in young adults with autism." Psychol Med. 2015 Mar;45(4):795-805. doi: 10.1017/S0033291714001858. Epub 2014 Aug 11.

Bieler, MD,Henry G., "Food Is Your Best Medicine", (1992)
Heritage Dr, John, "Notes on Microbial Infection for Medical Physicists", University of Leeds.
Coleman, John, "Protect Your Genes From Deadly Mutations", Life Extension, December 2009

Erejuwa OO, Gurtu S, Sulaiman SA, Ab Wahab MS, Sirajudeen KN, Salleh MS.," *Hypoglycemic and antioxidant effects of honey supplementation in streptozotocin-induced diabetic rats.*"
Int J Vitam Nutr Res. 2010 Jan;80(1):74-82. doi: 10.1024/0300-9831/a000008.

Erejuwa,, Omotayo O., Sulaiman, Siti A. , and Ab Wahab, Mohd S. "Honey - A Novel Antidiabetic Agent," Int J Biol Sci. 2012; 8(6): 913–934. Published online 2012 Jul 7. doi: 10.7150/ijbs.3697

Honey - A Novel Antidiabetic Agent
International Journal of Biological Sciences. 2012; 8(6)913

Gaschler[a], Michael M., Stockwell, Brent R. *"Lipid peroxidation in cell death"* Biochemical and Biophysical Research Communications
Volume 482, Issue 3, 15 January 2017, Pages 419-425

Girotti AW. J Lipid Res. "Lipid hydroperoxide generation, turnover, and effector action in biological systems",1998 Aug; 39(8):1529-42.

Howell, Dr. Edward, (1985), "Enzyme Nutrition: The Food Enzyme Concept".

Hume, E. Douglas "Pasteur or Beauchamp?", (C.W. Daniel Co. 1923, Reprint 1989)

Knize MG, Dolbeare FA, Cunningham PL, Felton JS. Princess Takamatsu "Mutagenic activity and heterocyclic amine content of the human diet" Symp. 1995; 23:30-8.

Martin, MD, William Coda (2003), "Dangers of Refined Sugar"

Molan, P.C.,B.Sc. Ph.D. (1998), "Honey as a Dressing for Wounds, Burns, and Ulcers: A Brief Review of Clinical Reports and Experimental Studies", Vol. 6, no. 4, Department of Biological Sciences, University of Waikato, Hamilton, New Zealand.

Mylonas C[1], Kouretas D. "Lipid peroxidation and tissue damage", In Vivo. 1999 May-Jun;13(3):295-309.

National Research Council (US) Committee on Diet, Nutrition, and Cancer, Washington (DC): National Academies Press (US); 1982.

Parplys AC[1], Petermann E, Petersen C, Dikomey E, Borgmann K. ,DNA damage by X-rays and their impact on replication processes. , Radiother Oncol. 2012 Mar;102(3):466-71.

Radiation Effects research Foundation, "How radiation harms cells",

Radoslav Goldman, Peter G. Shields, Food Mutagens, *The Journal of Nutrition*, Volume 133, Issue 3, March 2003, Pages 965S-973S,

Robbana-Barnat, Saida, Rabache, Maurice, Rialland, Emmanuelle, Fradin, Jacques, (1996), Heterocyclic Amines: Occurrence and Prevention in Cooked Food, Environmental Health Perspectives, Vol. 104, Number 3 Institut de Médecine Environnementale, Paris, France

Rona, MD, Zoltan P., "Rethinking Chlorinated Tap Water" and "Early Death comes From Drinking Distilled Water".

Rubin, Jordan S., (2003),"Patient Heal Thyself

Sugimura T[1], Wakabayashi K, Nakagama H, Nagao M. "Heterocyclic amines: Mutagens/carcinogens produced during cooking of meat and fish", Cancer Sci. 2004 Apr;95(4):290-9.

Sinha R[1], Kulldorff M, Chow WH, Denobile J, Rothman N., "Dietary intake of heterocyclic amines, meat-derived mutagenic activity, and risk of colorectal adenomas" Cancer Epidemiol Biomarkers Prev. 2001 May;10(5):559-62.

Sinha R, Chow WH, Kulldorff M, Denobile J, Butler J, Garcia-Closas M, Weil R, Hoover RN, Rothman N. "Well-done, grilled red meat increases the risk of colorectal adenomas",Cancer Res. 1999 Sep 1; 59(17):4320-4.

Sinha R[1], Rothman N, Brown ED, Salmon CP, Knize MG, Swanson CA, Rossi SC, Mark SD, Levander OA, Felton JS. "High concentrations of the carcinogen 2-amino-1-methyl-6-phenylimidazo- [4,5-b]pyridine (PhIP) occur in chicken but are dependent on the cooking method", <u>Cancer Res.</u> 1995 Oct 15;55(20):4516-9.

Sinclair, Ian, (1995) ,"Health: The Only Immunity".

Sulaiman SA, Mohamed M, , Sirajudeen KN, Jaafar H, *"Antioxidant protective effect of honey in cigarette smoke-induced testicular damage in rats."* Int J Mol Sci. 2011;12(9):5508-21.

Turesky RJ, Taylor J, Schnackenberg L, Freeman JP, Holland RD. J "Quantitation of carcinogenic heterocyclic aromatic amines and detection of novel heterocyclic aromatic amines in cooked meats and grill scrapings" Agric Food Chem. 2005 Apr 20; 53(8):3248-58.

Vikse R[1], Reistad R, Steffensen IL, Paulsen JE, Nyholm SH, Alexander J., "Heterocyclic amines in cooked meat" <u>Tidsskr Nor Laegeforen.</u> 1999 Jan 10;119(1):45-9.

Vonderplanitz, Aajonus, (2007),"We Want To Live", Los Angeles, CA: Carnelian Bay Castle Press.

Vonderplanitz, Aajonus, (2002), "The Recipe For Living Without Disease", Los Angeles, CA: Carnelian Bay Castle Press.

Wakabayashi K, Kim IS, Kurosaka R, Yamaizumi Z, Ushiyama H, Takahashi M, Koyota S, Tada A, Nukaya H, Goto S. Princess Takamatsu" Identification of new mutagenic heterocyclic amines and quantification of known heterocyclic amines", Symp. 1995; 23:39-49.

Wenner, Melinda, (Nov. 2007), "Humans carry more bacterial cells than human ones", Scientific America.

Young, Dr Robert, MD, (2001) "Sick and Tired".

THANK YOU

ABOUT THE AUTHOR

As a former competitive dancer, gymnast, and rhythmic gymnast, medical sales rep for some of the largest medical companies in the world, certified personal trainer, certified yoga teacher, health writer for the esteemed Aspen Healthy Planet magazine, host of the VoiceAmerica.com podcast "Raw To Radiant", pageant title holder, and mom......health and wellness has been part of my life. When my daughter was born with severe food allergies, I dove into studying nutrition and how the foods we eat either harm or heal the body.

In 2001, I created Idella's Natural Gourmet, one of the first gluten-free organic cookie companies that made delicious cookies for people with food allergies and sensitivities. I opened "Nur-ish ", an organic raw foods co-op that served delicious organic primal raw foods, and supported a local raw-dairy in the Aspen Colorado Valley, all the while committed to my daily yoga practice, volunteering at school, and raising a daughter.

I was born and raised in Flint, Michigan and have had the good fortune of not only living in various parts of our country learning western, eastern and alternative healing methods, but I have had life experiences that have exposed me to some of the best of the best. Currently, I work as a health coach, health researcher, author and speaker specializing in the detoxification and rebuilding of the physical body, the mind and our spirit.

Available for private, consultations and speaking engagements. Please contact directly for prices and availability. Kim@KimberlyLynnWilliams.com

THE DETOX BOX
If you are interested in information about a food box full of freshly made detoxifying foods, please email Kim. Kim@KimberlyLynnWilliams.com

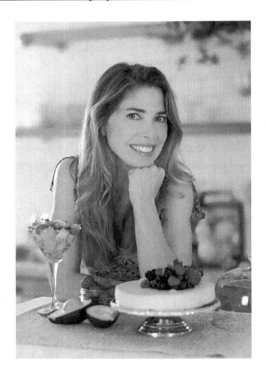

Made in the USA
Middletown, DE
03 November 2019

77810785R00099